ADHD...Now What?
How ADHD Coaching Can Help
You Take Back Your Power

of related interest

The Procrastination Playbook for Adults with ADHD
How to Catch Sneaky Forms of Procrastination Before They Catch You
Risa Williams
ISBN 978 1 80501 229 0
eISBN 978 1 80501 230 6

ADHD Girls to Women
Getting on the Radar
Lotta Borg Skoglund
ISBN 978 1 80501 054 8
eISBN 978 1 80501 055 5

We're All Neurodiverse
How to Build a Neurodiversity-Affirming Future
and Challenge Neuronormativity
Sonny Jane Wise
ISBN 978 1 83997 578 3
eISBN 978 1 83997 579 0

ADHD...
Now What?

How ADHD Coaching Can Help
You Take Back Your Power

KATIE FRIEDMAN
and **ALEX CAMPBELL**

Foreword by Lotta Borg Skoglund

Illustrated by Dan Edwards

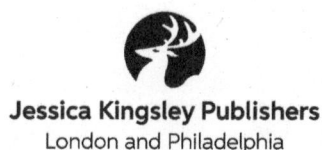

Jessica Kingsley Publishers
London and Philadelphia

First published in Great Britain in 2025 by Jessica Kingsley Publishers
An imprint of John Murray Press

1

Copyright © Katie Friedman and Alex Campbell 2025

The right of Katie Friedman and Alex Campbell to be identified as
the Author of the Work has been asserted by them in accordance
with the Copyright, Designs and Patents Act 1988.

Foreword © Lotta Borg Skoglund 2025

A CIP catalogue record for this title is available from the
British Library and the Library of Congress

ISBN 978 1 80501 766 0
eISBN 978 1 80501 767 7

Printed and bound in Great Britain by Clays Ltd

Jessica Kingsley Publishers' policy is to use papers that are natural,
renewable and recyclable products and made from wood grown in
sustainable forests. The logging and manufacturing processes are expected
to conform to the environmental regulations of the country of origin.

Jessica Kingsley Publishers
Carmelite House
50 Victoria Embankment
London EC4Y 0DZ

www.jkp.com

John Murray Press
Part of Hodder & Stoughton Ltd
An Hachette Company

The authorised representative in the EEA is Hachette Ireland, 8
Castlecourt Centre, Dublin 15, D15 XTP3, Ireland (email: info@hbgi.ie)

Dedicated to every ADHDer finding
their way back to themselves.

This book is for you.

Thanks

We would like to extend our heartfelt thanks to the following people and groups, whose contributions have been invaluable in bringing this book to life:

To our lived experience contributors – Your generosity in sharing your stories and the impact of ADHD coaching has been woven into the fabric of this book, bringing our words to life and offering a real-world perspective that will resonate with so many readers.

To Katie's partner, Phil, and their three boys, Byron, Mackenzie, and Gene – Thank you for allowing Katie the time to dedicate countless weekends to writing. Your support made it possible.

To Alex's partner, Millie, and their two kids, Tatum and Heath – We are so grateful for your patience during the late nights and early mornings as Alex worked with Katie across time zones to make this book a reality.

To Katie's mum – Thank you for your early proofreading and the hours you spent going through the manuscript with a fine-tooth comb, ensuring that the flow of the book was just right (or pointing out when it wasn't!).

To the Gold Mind Academy Faculty and students – Thank you for your bravery, especially during the early pilot days of our training. You've taught us so much about ADHD coaching and its impact, and this book is richer for it.

To all our coaching clients – Thank you for teaching us what is most beneficial and important in ADHD coaching. Your insights have helped shape the approach we present in this book.

To Lotta Borg Skoglund – We are deeply grateful for your generosity in reading and writing the foreword. Your contribution has set the perfect tone for this book.

To Dan Edwards – Thank you for your last-minute brilliance in creating the beautiful illustrations that bring our ideas to life. You turned our mumbled words into visual clarity, and we are so appreciative of your hard work.

To Sean Townsend at Jessica Kingsley Publishers – Thank you for your patience, guidance, and countless Zoom calls and emails. Your editorial expertise has been invaluable in shaping this book into what it is today.

To each other – We've learned so much about ourselves, our ADHD, and how to live authentically as ADHDers in a world not designed for us. Writing this book together, despite the challenges of being on opposite sides of the world (with Alex in New Zealand and Katie in the UK), has been a testament to the power of collaboration and shared vision.

To YOU, our reader – Thank you for picking up a copy of our book, and if you're an ADHDer, for bothering to read this bit! Now, go ahead and dive into the contents page. Start with whatever part interests you most. We hope you find yourself and feel truly seen within the pages of this book. Enjoy!

CONTENTS

Foreword

Attention deficit hyperactivity disorder (ADHD) is a complex neurodevelopmental condition affecting millions of individuals worldwide. While evidence-based medical treatments like medication and therapeutic approaches play a crucial role in managing ADHD, there is growing recognition of the value of ADHD coaching as a complementary approach to support those with ADHD in reaching their full potential.

Living with ADHD in a society tailored for neurotypicals can be a life of both challenges and hidden potential. Traditional approaches focusing on what's wrong with your ADHD brain rather than unfolding ways to thrive and grow alongside your ADHD are increasingly being challenged as we understand more and more about the complex human brain and neurodiversity.

This is a comprehensive book about ADHD coaching – what it is, how it works, and the transformative impact it can have. The authors, Katie Friedman and Alex Campbell, draw on their own extensive experience as ADHD coaches and coach trainers to offer an insightful exploration of this emerging field. They also generously share their own ADHD experiences and how personalized ADHD coaching was the missing piece of the puzzle for them.

In this book, you will learn how ADHD coaching can be tailored to your unique needs and challenges. The focus is set on self-discovery, strengths-based approaches, and actionable steps for personal growth.

It is clear that the authors know their audience well. So well, in fact, that they decided to switch up the usual order of the chapters, knowing that many of us ADHD readers tend to flip straight to the end of a book or manual before starting from the beginning. Embracing the spirit of spontaneity that often accompanies ADHD, they structured the content to be flexible and engaging no matter where you start reading. Because who says you need to follow a linear path when learning about ADHD?

I strongly recommend this book since it has long been clear to me, as a representative of psychiatry and healthcare, that ADHD coaching can be an attractive and cost-effective complement to traditional ADHD care and self-care. Whether you're new to the concept of ADHD coaching or have long struggled with neurodivergent challenges, this book serves as a compassionate guide to help you not just survive, but thrive. By supporting real-life skill-building, ADHD coaching helps bridge the gap that Professor Russell Barkley MD PhD so elegantly described: ADHD is not about knowing what to do – but about doing what you know!

Lotta Borg Skoglund MD PhD

Introduction: Setting the ADHD Scene

WHY THIS BOOK MATTERS

So you've got ADHD. And you've finally found the courage to talk about it. What's the reaction? Often, it goes something like this: 'Yeah, but aren't we all a little bit ADHD?'

It's true that the explosion in ADHD awareness and support has been significant, and is influenced by several critical factors (Abdelnour, Jansen, & Gold, 2022), including a broadening of the diagnostic criteria to allow more individuals to be identified.

However, in reality 'we are all a bit ADHD' trivializes your ADHD; a difference that, as you know all too well, presents real and significant challenges.

So how do we change this? How can we cultivate a deeper, more accurate understanding of ADHD – both for you, the ADH-Der, and also for society at large?

One of the most powerful tools we have is professional ADHD coaching.

For years, the only things I ever thought about myself were bad. I was a disappointment 'at best', and at worst, I was where potential essentially went to die. I felt different in the sense that I felt less than everyone else, but often as a result of problems they thought could be easily solved with things like 'concentrating', being 'nicer', acting more like 'everyone else', and the big one, 'putting more effort in'.

But I was trying so much harder than anyone else could even see.

Finding out I had ADHD helped me to understand why I was having these experiences, and was really validating... but on its own, it somehow changes everything and nothing, all at the same time. Because the same things were still hard. And knowing why didn't change that.

But something did, and that was ADHD coaching.

SUZY JACKSON, THE TECHNICOLOUR PROJECT,
ADHD SPECIALIST COACH

WHY IS A COACHING APPROACH SO IMPORTANT FOR INDIVIDUALS WITH ADHD?

Coaching, rooted in the principles of positive psychology, significantly shifts the focus from 'what's wrong' with us to 'what's right' with us. Unlike traditional psychological methods that often pathologize issues, coaching believes that we are inherently capable and do not require fixing. Coaching empowers us to use our own strengths and insights, making it an indispensable approach in the discovery and understanding of ADHD.

> My brain is as unique to me as my fingerprint, and I'm also fiercely independent and like to work things out for myself... which, really, is what I get from ADHD coaching. A string of surprises; things that I say that I didn't know I knew, but that were in there somewhere, coaxed out with some clever questioning and a safe place for me to examine the parts of my brain, and myself, that I never really knew how to use.
>
> **SUZY JACKSON, THE TECHNICOLOUR PROJECT, ADHD SPECIALIST COACH**

While medical professionals are crucial for diagnosis and treatment, they often lack the capacity to engage deeply with the nuanced and situational daily realities faced by us ADHDers. In contrast, ADHD coaches spend extensive time with clients, offering safe spaces to explore what it truly means to thrive as an ADHDer. ADHD coaches often have a first-hand understanding of the challenges and strengths involved, enabling them to provide more empathetic and nuanced support.

Starting my ADHD coaching was a transformative experience. Finally having someone to talk to who understood what it was like to live with ADHD was incredible. It was the first time I felt truly seen and heard as a woman with ADHD, without any need for masking or fear of judgement. For once, someone was taking me seriously, and that alone was life-changing.

NIKKI HARDY, ADHD CAREER COACH

INTERSECTIONALITY

In Nikki's quote above, she talks about being heard as a woman with ADHD. When discussing ADHD and neurodiversity, it is crucial to incorporate the concept of intersectionality, developed by lawyer and Black Feminist, Kimberlé Crenshaw, in 1989. Intersectionality recognizes that individuals experience discrimination uniquely, based on the interconnection of multiple social categorizations such as race, gender, age, socio-economic status, and disability. We are never navigating just ADHD but will have other identity markers that are important to us in the context of ADHD. We are likely to feel these parts of our identity more if we are proud of them and/or because we are marginalized in systems of privilege. Which identity markers feel important to you and your ADHD experience?

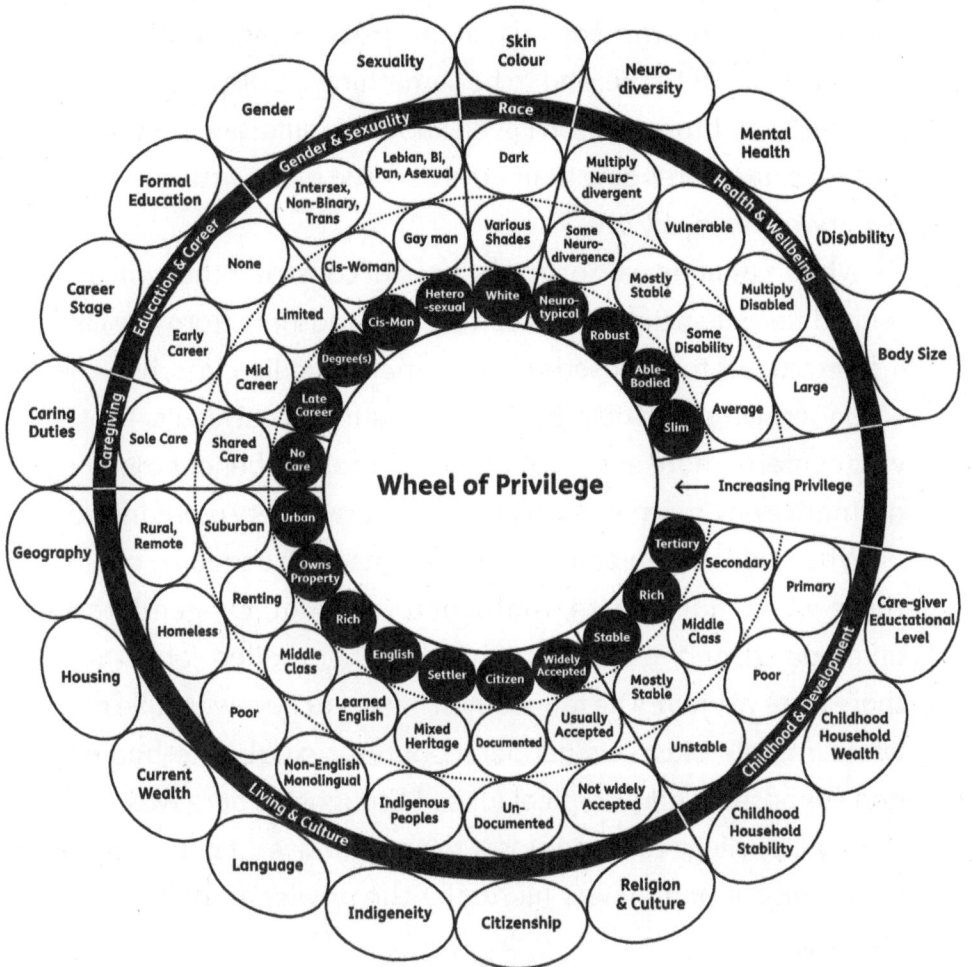

Figure I.1: The Intersectionality Wheel

Source: Adapted from the Academic Wheel of Privilege (FORRT, 2023), which builds on Sylvia Duckworth's Wheel of Power/Privilege (2020) and the original conception of intersectionality by Kimberlé Crenshaw (1989). Adaptation © 2024 by Gold Mind Academy.

WHAT IS NORMAL?

'You're too much/too loud/too quiet/not quite right' – many of us have received messaging that we don't fit in or that we are not 'normal'. This messaging can be direct or very subtle. This may have led us to pretend to be something we are not in order to fit in. Sometimes we don't even know the difference between when we are pretending to fit in, are scared of not fitting in or of being who we really are.

What is defined as 'normal' is a social construct that will differ in different societies and cultures. For authors from the UK, 'normal' tends to be based on white, male, middle-class, heterosexual, cis-gendered able-bodied, and neurotypical ideals. Those who conform more easily to what is normal will benefit more in normative environments which reflect how society is organized.

When I was in senior leadership teams in an academy chain, there were more white, male, heterosexual, cis-gendered, able-bodied, and neurotypical headteachers called 'John' than there were women. The few women headteachers were like me; white, middle-class, cis-gendered, heterosexual, able-bodied, and supposedly neurotypical (or so I thought!). There was very clearly a privilege to being closer to a normative, and further up the organizational power hierarchy, the privilege was increasingly normative.

Hierarchies, recruitment procedures, expectations, and organizational cultures will privilege a normative person because of cognitive bias, whether we realize it or not. We have all received messaging that normatives are 'better' through representation in culture, media, family, schools, and workplaces, which prize normative ways of being. We internalize these messages, whether they reinforce our privilege or go directly against who we are. Just because we identify as having ADHD doesn't mean we haven't internalized that being disabled is 'less than' – that is, we have internalized ableism.

The same can be true for all systems of power. If we are more marginalized there will be more internalizing of 'less than', and the layers of 'who I pretend to be' and 'who I am scared I am' get thicker and often more confused. This is why pathologizing terms like 'imposter syndrome' where a person doesn't feel as if they belong or are worthy are so problematic. The term suggests that this is a problem with the individual and one they must overcome rather than a problem with the way the system marginalizes the individual. Internalized negativity works to isolate us and make us feel as if we are alone and ashamed and more disempowered. If we are more marginalized, we will be swimming harder to survive in these systems. If we benefit from them, they act like invisible floats that we don't necessarily feel.

Those of us who experience more marginalization will experience more compromised safety and less choice, certainty, and clarity. This leads to hiding difference (as Nikki mentions in the need for masking above) or feeling bad about being different (as we can see in Suzy's story above). If the aim of coaching is to enable empowerment – which we believe it is – we need to become discerning about environments and systems and how they impact on us.

We will also have to examine how we have internalized marginalization as a problem within as well as a problem with our environment. Sadly, not only do we internalize where we may be the problem, we also internalize the system of othering and become the environment for others. We internalize racist, sexist, ableist, classist, and homophobic ideas.

PROFESSIONALIZATION OF NON-CLINICAL ADHD SUPPORT

For many of us who have been privileged to access support, it has been the norm to encounter support that is well intentioned yet ineffective because brain wiring differences have not been understood by the helpers (see examples in Katie and Alex's stories below). With the 'explosion' of ADHD awareness and diagnosis, the need for the professionalization of support mechanisms – including ADHD coaching – has never been greater. Therefore, our commitment in this book is to illuminate how tailored, professional coaching can genuinely fit the unique strengths and challenges of your ADHD. This professionalization isn't merely about enhancing standards. It's about ensuring that ADHD coaching is a transformative force, empowering us through high-quality, reliable support.

THE AUTHORS

Katie

The first time I ever considered that my brain might be different was when a fellow member of the senior leadership team said she thought she was autistic. This brave act of normalizing neurodiversity in a normative school culture sparked my curiosity, but I was speeding way too fast to really catch it. Sadly, it wasn't until I crashed out of my school leadership career four months later that my journey to discover myself, including my neurodivergence, began.

Along the way, as I tried to recover from burnout, I experienced 'help' that didn't serve me effectively because my counsellor and coaches seemed to have no understanding of ADHD or how it affected me and intersected with my other identities. For example, when they used Gestalt techniques where they shared how they were experiencing me (as speedy and stress inducing) in order to raise my awareness of how I was feeling, I experienced intense rejection and began behaving differently (masking) to be safe – people pleasing while paying for it, if you will! When discussing my parents and their impact on me, we couldn't discuss their neurodivergence.

When we discussed my addiction to coffee, the steer seemed to be simply about giving it up rather than understanding this was effectively me 'self-medicating' to manage my energy. In the end, I challenged them and said they would need more training to work with clients like me.

On the one hand, assertively challenging in this vulnerable space was very empowering. The counsellor, to their credit, responded with love and humility. 'I think you are going to change the world,' they said. In my head I thought, 'Watch me'.

I have carried their words with me ever since but it took me six months to realize that the support wasn't serving me and this delayed my recovery and caused unnecessary frustration, isolation, and shame. Eventually, my belief that I could trust people to help me was so eroded, I decided to learn my way out of burnout by becoming the coach I needed. After extensive coach training, I realized this was a specialist ADHD coach.

During my 162 hours of extra ADHD coach training, I met Alex and we started to discuss our approach to ADHD coaching based on what we were learning and experiencing (and what we weren't learning or experiencing!). We decided that our education and psychotherapy backgrounds, along with the different strengths we had, were a complementary blend for our coach training company Gold Mind Academy.

In 2023, I attended the ADHD world conference in Amsterdam. I wandered over to one of the organizers responsible for evaluation and said the best way to improve the conference would be to ask any ADHDer. Our creative solution-focused brains would nuance all kinds of inclusive tweaks to the event that would benefit all (including the many clinicians whom I suspect were neurodivergent themselves). I was told that there was a form I could fill in but that today and tomorrow were not really 'for' me and that 'patients' day was on the final morning'. In this very disempowering moment, I thought, 'Watch me'.

I appreciate that this defiant response is thanks to my ADHD and my intersecting privilege and marginalization in this space: I am white, middle class, and have parents who worked in academia so I wasn't short on expectation or economic means to achieve when growing up. My marginalization as a middle-aged woman with ADHD in that conference full of majority white, middle-class clinicians and academics was my choice to disclose. Having been a leader in education with several degrees and qualifications, and an organizer of events for over 15 years, it was farcical and indeed a privilege to only suddenly have to experience this ableism in midlife. I immediately saw the bigger picture; ableism getting in the way of effective precision health that was questionably the purpose of the conference. I saw the need for what the disability rights movement has been preaching since the 1970s: 'nothing about us without us'.

We don't need to be saved or fixed; we need to be included and empowered to speak up and we will have to bring our own seats to the table. The ADHD coaching I have had intermittently over the last three years has helped me to do this. That's why Alex and I are on a mission to make ADHD coaching the best it can be to serve the widest range of ADHDers effectively. We hope this book will demystify this important support.

Alex

People often say that being diagnosed with ADHD at four in 1990 must have been a privilege. In some ways, it was. I fit the typical ADHD demographic of the early 90s – a cis white boy in private education, the very group most research focused on. But the stigma around my ADHD was profound and often used more as a weapon than support. My time at boarding school was a mixed experience. While I benefitted from small class sizes and more personal attention, the competitive, cliquish environment left me feeling isolated. The narrative I internalized was that my ADHD was a problem, something broken in me, and the 'support' I received – whether from educators, friends, or family – often reinforced that feeling. It taught me to make myself smaller, to avoid drawing attention to my struggles, and to not need support.

I vividly recall being pulled from a Spanish class I loved at the age of ten for extra English lessons due to my dyslexia. While the school meant well, it had a devastating impact on my self-esteem. Spanish was something I enjoyed, and being removed from it felt like a punishment. The focus on 'important' subjects like English left me feeling incapable in one of the areas of my life that brought me some confidence. This was a classic example of well-intentioned help that did more harm than good.

When I was 15, my doctors switched me from Ritalin to a new stimulant medication, promising fewer side effects. Instead, I quickly became depressed and more anxious than before. I was also seeing a therapist at the time, supposedly to help with my mental health challenges. Yet, despite my ADHD diagnosis being known, it was never addressed in therapy. I remember sitting through sessions, watching the clock, or asking to leave the room just to escape. I often thought, 'Why am I even here? Nothing's helping.' The therapy missed the mark entirely because it failed to consider my ADHD.

In my late twenties, I started working with a psychodynamic therapist, who helped me recognize the importance of environments that suited my way of working. But even then, ADHD didn't feature in our conversations. I had internalized the idea that I had outgrown it – an idea my psychiatrist supported. Now, I see this as internalized ableism, both on my part and theirs. I spent too long in therapy, not because I needed it, but because I couldn't figure out how to end the relationship – a classic ADHD tendency to people-please.

It wasn't until I was re-diagnosed during my psychotherapy training that I began to accept my ADHD again. This re-diagnosis brought a wave of insights, but it still shocks me that neurodiversity was never once mentioned during my entire five years of training. That gap eventually led me to coaching. At first, I entered the world of coaching with a chip on my shoulder, thinking I was better because of my years of therapy training. But then I realized coaching was what had been missing all along. It wasn't about fixing what was wrong with me – it was about finding what was right.

When I met Katie, we spent a year blending our approaches

to ADHD coaching, and that's how Gold Mind was born. Our partnership has taught me what true support looks like. Being vulnerable about my ADHD, sharing my overwhelm and feelings of inadequacy, owning my natural strengths, has been a mirror for the support I want to offer my clients. Trusting Katie and witnessing her own vulnerabilities has made me realize that the kind of nurturing, supportive environment we've built in Gold Mind is what ADHD coaching should be for everyone.

WHO IS THIS BOOK AIMED AT?

This book is framed with YOU, ADHD adults, in mind. You may be a late discoverer of ADHD or perhaps diagnosed as a child but have not yet experienced tailored support.

If we are neurodivergent, we are more likely than not to qualify for multiple and overlapping co-occurrences such as autism, dyslexia, dyspraxia, Tourette's, and bipolar disorder, whether diagnosed or not. For example, if we qualify for an ADHD diagnosis, research indicates there is a 50–60% chance we would also qualify for an autistic diagnosis (Joshi *et al.*, 2017; Zablotsky, Bramlett, & Blumberg, 2020). Similarly, among those diagnosed as autistic, studies suggest there is an 80% chance the individual would also meet the criteria for ADHD (Young *et al.*, 2020). Despite this significant overlap, the medical system tends to treat these labels as distinct, which is more profitable, but creates barriers to a deeper understanding of ourselves and our unique neurodivergence.

For the purpose of this book, we will concentrate on the ADHD traits; however, our models and style of coaching work with all types of neurodivergence and will need to be adapted to the individual and unique expression of ADHD.

For far too many of us, ADHD diagnosis (or any other diagnosis) – let alone ADHD coaching – is unknown, inaccessible, and unaffordable. Some of us avoid engaging in coaching because the idea of giving up time for a reward which is unclear does not seem worth it. For some, not knowing that tailored ADHD coaching even exists means that we have spent huge sums of money seeking help, which all too often ends up with us feeling as if we've failed; the reason that nothing has changed is 'on us'.

You may be unclear about what ADHD coaching is and how it can help. After a lifetime of not understanding yourself and trying to live up to normative expectations, you may bring this with you to coaching in the hope of a quick fix. The goals we set for ourselves are often unrealistic and ableist; wanting to solve or fix our disability with some 'tools, tips, and tricks'.

This book aims to highlight the need for ADHD coaching, its value, and the practicalities of getting well-qualified support, as well as sources of funding. We hope that the interweaved lived experiences of navigating without support and with support will resonate with you and you will be inspired and clear about what is possible.

HOW TO USE THIS BOOK AND WHAT WILL I GET OUT OF EACH CHAPTER?

This book has been written with ADHDers in mind, and we are fully aware that the journey through the following pages may well not be linear. We think that there is merit in reading each chapter and will set out our reasons below. While some might say that it is advisable to follow the book's structure, we know that ADHDers don't do well with being told! Given the ADHDer tendency to start at the end, we thought we would begin with the end in mind here:

- Chapter 4: What is the Impact of ADHD Coaching?

  This chapter presents testimonials and insights from those who have experienced the benefits of ADHD coaching. It examines the process of change and its positive impacts, highlighting how micro shifts can lead to thriving with ADHD. This chapter is worth reading to really understand what can change as a result of ADHD coaching.

- Chapter 3: Getting Started with an ADHD Coach

  This chapter covers the practicalities of ADHD coaching. It includes details on funding ADHD coaching, provides guidance on selecting the best coach, and explains the commitment required. This chapter also explores how to maximize the coaching experience, addresses when coaching might not be the right approach, and considers life beyond ADHD coaching, including the concept of self-coaching. This chapter is worth reading in order to navigate your next steps to getting ADHD coaching.

- Chapter 2: What is ADHD Coaching and How Does it Work?

  This chapter delves into the nature of ADHD coaching and

its impact on individuals. It covers the fundamentals of ADHD coaching, exploring key concepts such as the ADHD lens, narrative change, strengths-based approaches, and the importance of emotional granularity. It also discusses how to put these concepts together to live purposefully with ADHD.

- Chapter 1: What is ADHD and How is it Experienced?

  This chapter sets the stage by discussing the significance of understanding ADHD in a broader context. Key concepts include the explosion in ADHD awareness, executive functions, sensory differences, and the ADHD brain's unique wiring. It also examines intersectionality, the connection between ADHD and trauma, and the challenges of living in a world not designed for neurodivergent individuals.

The stories within this book, including those of Katie and Alex, are diverse. By highlighting these differences, an intersectional lens is applied to understanding ADHD and obtaining support. ADHD affects people differently depending on how close or far they are from normative expectations and privilege. The phrase, 'if you've met one ADHDer, you've only met one ADHDer,' encapsulates this variability.

At the end of each of the four chapters of this book, there is a 'summary' that breaks down the key takeaways from that chapter; there are also reflective questions to help you personalize what you have read. These questions are designed to help you delve deeper into what might be important to you from that chapter.

They aim to aid you in understanding your own ADHD and in gaining clarity on how you might approach ADHD coaching.

KEY TERMS AND MODELS

This list of terms and models will help you understand the language, key terms of phrase, and coaching models used in this book. You can use this as a point to refer back to at any time you are unsure of words used.

ACC & PCC Credentialed Coach (International Coaching Federation, 2024): ACC stands for Associate Certified Coach, and PCC stands for Professional Certified Coach. These refer to the level of credentialing a coach has reached. For the International Coaching Federation, the first level of accreditation is Associate Coach Credentialed (ACC). In order to attain this level, a coach must reach a minimum of 60 hours of coach training and at least 100 hours of coaching experience. To reach the level of Professional Coach Credential (PCC), they must complete more than 125 hours of coach training and at least 500 coaching hours.

Ableism/Ableist (a term first used by US feminists in the 1980s; Council of the London Borough of Haringey, 1986): Discrimination, prejudice, or social prejudice against people with disabilities or neurodivergent conditions. It manifests in attitudes, actions, and systems that devalue and limit the potential of individuals with disabilities or neurodivergence.

Attention stimulus (commonly used in recent psychology literature): Any factor or input that captures and holds an individual's focus and concentration. This can include sensory inputs, emotional triggers, or engaging activities that effectively draw and sustain attention.

Being 'in drama' (Karpman, 1968): When someone occupies one of the roles on the Drama Triangle – Victim, Persecutor, or Rescuer – and may or may not be aware of their participation in these dysfunctional interactions. This state often perpetuates conflict and hinders effective communication and resolution.

Character strengths (Peterson & Seligman, 2004): The positive traits or capacities that exist within all individuals and are essential for well-being and personal growth. Identified through extensive psychological research, the Values in Action (VIA) Classification outlines 24 universal strengths, such as kindness, creativity, and resilience, which are grouped under six broader virtues: wisdom, courage, humanity, justice, temperance, and transcendence. These strengths provide a foundation for thriving and can be cultivated through intentional practice.

Class system (Weber, 1946): A form of social stratification where individuals and groups are divided into hierarchical categories based on factors such as wealth, income, education, and occupation. The class system tends to reproduce itself, with people often remaining in the class into which they are born, reinforcing inequality and access to resources.

Drama and Winning Triangle (Karpman, 1968): The Drama

Triangle outlines dysfunctional interaction roles: Victim, Persecutor, and Rescuer. The Winning Triangle, proposed as an alternative response to being 'in drama', promotes empowered interactions with roles such as Thrive (instead of Victim), Challenger (instead of Persecutor), and Coach (instead of Rescuer).

Emotional regulation (adapted from recent psychology literature): The ability to manage and respond to one's emotional experiences effectively. It involves recognizing, understanding, and adjusting one's emotions in a way that helps navigate various situations and interactions.

Executive functions (Brown, 2024): Cognitive processes that serve as the brain's management system, enabling individuals to plan, focus attention, remember instructions, and manage multiple tasks effectively. These skills include working memory, flexible thinking, and self-control.

Flow state (Csíkszentmihályi, 1990): When someone is so involved in a specific task or activity that nothing else around them appears to matter. This can be likened to the term 'hyperfocus'.

Gaslighting (adapted from psychological abuse literature, coined by Patrick Hamilton in his 1938 play *Gas Light*): A form of psychological manipulation where a person or group causes someone to doubt their own perceptions, memories, or reality. This tactic is often used to gain control or power over the individual, leading them to question their own sanity or judgement.

Global North and Global South: Terms used to describe the economic, political, and social divide between more and less economically developed regions of the world. They were popularized in the 1970s and 1980s, particularly in discussions of global economic development, as alternatives to terms like 'First World' and 'Third World'. The shift aimed to move away from the Cold War era of ideological framing. These terms emerged from the works of economists, political scientists, and sociologists who were studying global inequalities and development.

Heteronormativity (Warner, 1993): The belief that heterosexuality is the default, natural, or normal mode of sexual orientation, which reinforces traditional gender roles and marginalizes non-heterosexual identities and relationships. This concept underpins social institutions, policies, and cultural norms that privilege heterosexuality and stigmatize LGBTQ+ individuals.

Hidden Disability Sunflower Lanyard: A discreet symbol used by people with hidden disabilities, such as autism, ADHD, or chronic conditions, to signal to staff and others that they may require additional support, assistance, or understanding. It was first introduced in the UK in 2016 at airports but has since expanded to supermarkets, public transport, and other venues. Wearing the lanyard is voluntary and helps to raise awareness about disabilities that are not immediately visible.

Hyperfocus (commonly used in recent ADHD literature): Intense and sustained concentration on a specific task or activity,

INTRODUCTION: SETTING THE ADHD SCENE

often to the exclusion of everything else. This state can lead to high productivity.

Intersectionality (Crenshaw, 1989): A framework for understanding how various aspects of a person's social and political identities (such as race, gender, disability, and class) intersect and create overlapping systems of discrimination or disadvantage. It highlights that individuals may face multiple, interconnected forms of oppression simultaneously.

Late diagnosis (commonly used in recent ADHD literature): The identification and confirmation of a neurodivergent condition, such as ADHD, in an individual over 16 years of age. This often comes after years of coping with unexplained challenges and can lead to a reassessment of one's personal and professional experiences.

Masking (Hull *et al.*, 2017): The conscious or unconscious suppression of neurodivergent traits or behaviours in order to fit into societal norms or expectations. It often involves mimicking neurotypical behaviours, hiding difficulties, or downplaying differences to avoid stigma or social rejection. While masking can be a coping mechanism, it can also lead to exhaustion, anxiety, and a loss of personal authenticity over time. It is particularly common in individuals with ADHD and autism.

Medical/Deficit model (adapted from early 20th-century medical literature): This views neurodivergent conditions as disorders or deficits that need to be diagnosed, treated, cured, or fixed. It focuses on the limitations and challenges associated with these conditions rather than their potential strengths or positive aspects.

Model of Self (Ditzler, 2003): This model, by coach Jinny Ditzler, separates self-identity into three layers: the outer layer is 'Who I pretend to be', representing the facade or persona shown to the world; the middle layer is 'Who I'm scared I am', reflecting fears and insecurities about one's true nature; and the core layer is 'Who I really am', which embodies the authentic self, free from pretences and fears.

Neurodiverse (used in the autistic self-advocacy community, Singer, 1998): Describes the natural variation in all human brains and promotes the value of diversity in neurological functioning; it is not a term used to describe a single individual.

Neurodivergent/Neurodivergence (Asasumasu, 2000): Refers to individuals whose neurological development and functioning differ from what is considered typical or neurotypical. This term encompasses a range of conditions such as ADHD, autism, dyslexia, and dyspraxia.

Neurotypical (used in the autistic self-advocacy community, Singer, 1998): Refers to individuals whose neurological development and functioning align with what is considered typical or standard in society.

Neuronormativity (Walker, 2014; used in the autistic self-advocacy groups from the 2000s): Refers to the societal and cultural assumption that neurotypical (non-neurodivergent) ways of thinking, behaving, and processing information are the default or superior norms. This concept critiques how social structures and institutions cater to neurotypical individuals while marginalizing or pathologizing neurodivergent ways of being. Neuronormativity is often upheld by medical models of disability and is a key target of neurodiversity advocacy, which seeks to challenge and expand what is considered 'normal' in society.

Normative systems (Durkheim, 1895): Frameworks of rules, values, and behaviours considered 'normal' or acceptable in a society or group. These systems enforce conformity and can marginalize those who do not fit within these established norms. In relation to neurodiversity, normative systems perpetuate neuronormativity, reinforcing social biases that favour neurotypical behaviour and marginalize neurodivergent individuals.

Patriarchy (hooks, 2000; Walby, 1990): Refers to a social system in which men hold primary power, dominating in roles of political leadership, moral authority, social privilege, and control over property. Patriarchy reinforces gender roles that subordinate women and non-binary individuals, while elevating men to positions of power.

Pedestalling (adapted from recent coaching literature): In the context of coaching, refers to elevating a coach to an idealized status, viewing them as an expert. This can create unrealistic expectations and hinder the collaborative nature of the coaching relationship, potentially impacting the client's self-efficacy and growth.

Rejection sensitivity (commonly used in recent ADHD literature): An increased vulnerability to perceiving and strongly reacting to rejection or criticism, often resulting in heightened emotional distress.

Self-diagnosis (commonly used in recent neurodiversity literature): When an individual identifies and acknowledges their own neurodivergent condition, such as ADHD, based on personal research and self-reflection. This can occur before, or in place of, a formal diagnosis from a medical professional.

Situational variability (Kirby & Smith, 2021): The fluctuation in an individual's behaviour, performance, or abilities depending on the context or environment. This concept recognizes that these variables depend on the TIE model: Task, Individual, and Environment, which together influence how someone functions at any given time.

Social model (Oliver, 1983): Views neurodivergent conditions as differences rather than deficits, emphasizing that societal barriers and lack of accommodations create challenges for individuals. It advocates for changes in society to remove these barriers and promote inclusion and accessibility.

Spiky profile (Doyle, 2022): A pattern of cognitive strengths and challenges where an individual exhibits a significant disparity between their abilities. Common in neurodivergent individuals, it highlights exceptional skills in certain areas alongside notable challenges in others, contrasting with a more evenly distributed neurotypical cognitive skill set.

Titration (commonly used in recent medical literature): The process of adjusting the dosage of a medication to find the optimal therapeutic level. This is done gradually to balance effectiveness while minimizing side effects.

Time perception differences (Time blindness) (commonly used in recent ADHD literature): Often referred to as time blindness, this refers to variations in how individuals perceive the passage of time as either 'now' or 'not now'. These differences can influence one's ability to manage time, meet deadlines, and plan for future tasks/events.

White supremacy (Coates, 2015): The belief or ideology that white people are superior to people of other racial backgrounds, and should therefore dominate society. This concept often manifests in both overt and systemic ways, reinforcing racial hierarchies that privilege white individuals over people of colour. White supremacy has deep historical roots, tied to colonialism, slavery, and segregation.

What is ADHD and How is it Experienced?

In this chapter, we aim to unravel the complexities of ADHD, providing a holistic understanding that goes beyond the conventional medical perspective. Here, we'll explore a comprehensive view of ADHD – both the neurobiological differences and the impact of navigating systems that are not designed for these often unknown differences. We refer to this as a resulting survival mode.

While you probably have a comprehensive understanding of the neurobiological differences and traits of ADHD, we encourage you to read this chapter to deepen your clarity on how survival mode may be impacting you. We believe that with clarity and certainty comes choice and we hope that you will become aware of new ways of being which can be imagined and implemented with ADHD coaching.

We'll argue that finding out is only the beginning and that ADHD coaching can help you shift from *surviving* to *thriving*.

As a first step in this shift, it is important to be explicit about the medical model of understanding ADHD and how this may be a barrier to thriving with ADHD. We advocate for an integrated psychosocial model for understanding how ADHD really works given the situational nature of ADHD as a disability.

THE MEDICAL AND SOCIAL MODELS OF DISABILITY

Understanding the medical model

The medical model of disability views disabilities primarily as a problem of the person, directly caused by disease, trauma, or other health conditions, which requires medical care provided in the form of individual treatment by professionals. This is clearly seen in the American Medical Association's *Journal of Ethics* (2016):

> The medical model focuses on curing or managing illness or disability. By extension, the medical model supposes a compassionate or just society invests resources in health care and related services in an attempt to cure or manage disabilities medically. This is in an aim to expand or improve functioning, and to allow disabled people to lead a more 'normal' life.

In the context of ADHD, the medical model tends to focus on the deficits and ways to mitigate symptoms through medication and other clinical interventions (Brown, 2004). This approach can often lead to a pathologizing perspective, one in which ADHD can be seen as something 'wrong' with the individual that needs to be 'cured', 'managed', or 'fixed'.

Unfortunately, this ableist perspective means that the helping professions are invited into disempowering saviour-type approaches, which in turn can be deeply damaging to those that are trying to seek help from them. This culture of ableism, where difference means deficit, is sadly a barrier to self-discovery of neurodivergence and safety among helping professionals and clinicians themselves. Instead, medical professionals who are also neurodivergent themselves, but don't yet realize it, inadvertently distance themselves from neurodivergence or dismiss and minimize it in themselves and, in turn, those who come to them for help.

Another reason why many neurodivergent professionals don't see themselves as neurodivergent is that the medical model is based on the white male experience. Here Pippa Simou reflects on how close she was to ADHD in education and home and still couldn't see herself as neurodivergent and the impact this had on her ability to support others:

I was consumed with the question 'How could I have worked in education, been a parent of an ADHD child, supported other parents in the same situation, delivered training to professionals AND still not know about how ADHD might show up for girls and women?' Although as a teacher I did know what ADHD stood for, I had no idea of the nature and many 'faces' of this condition. I received no specific training and did not seek any myself.

The extent of my ADHD educational support knowledge was 'give them some blu·tack' and keep it 'pacy'! The thought that I had been teaching 'younger me' and would have perpetuated this damaging experience, unintentional though it was, left a mark on me.

PIPPA SIMOU, CHARTERED COACHING PSYCHOLOGIST
AND ADHD-INFORMED COACH

Pippa goes on to discuss her ableism; that being a 'professional', a 'teacher', and a 'parent' meant it wasn't possible to have a hidden disability. These hierarchical roles assume a 'helper' or 'power over' perspective, which means it is harder to see ourselves as having our own needs.

Here Lynne Tapper (a former NHS professional and parent to neurodivergent children) talks about her resistance to getting support:

'What's stopping you from getting an ADHD assessment?'

It was a challenge and I could feel resistance within me. I realized that I had a belief that it was okay for other people to be different but it wasn't okay for me. I could happily support others but I didn't need or want any of that kind of support for myself.

Through raising an autistic child, whose ways of processing and perceiving information were so different to my own, I had developed a strong neurotypical identity. This challenge to reconsider my identity initially felt like a threat. It got me thinking hard and helped me realize that I needed to find out whether or not I had ADHD for two reasons:

1. To gain a better and deeper understanding of who I am and how I tick.
2. To begin the process of understanding and accepting the differences in myself and as a result more fully embrace differences in others.

LYNNE TAPPER, NEURODIVERSITY COACH

Lynne shows how internalized ableism, perpetuated by the medical model around us, can get in the way of exploring who we are and, in turn, how we show up for others.

The social model of disability and ADHD

Contrasting sharply with the medical model, the social model of disability argues that disability is caused by the way society is organized, rather than by a person's impairment or difference. It looks at ways of removing barriers that restrict life choices for disabled people (Oliver, 1990). For you, the ADHDer, this model shifts the focus from fixing you to modifying the societal environment and structures to accommodate diverse neurological profiles. This approach underlines the importance of understanding ADHD not just in terms of challenges, but also considering the societal barriers that exacerbate these challenges. These societal barriers may be more or less depending on the level of marginalization or privilege an ADHDer holds in relation to social systems of power.

ADHD coaching and the social model

Aligned with the social model, ADHD coaching does not seek to 'fix' you but rather to empower you to understand your unique neurological makeup and how it interacts with environments and power systems which privilege a normative society. This type of coaching is pivotal in helping you identify how societal norms and expectations impact you and in exploring strategies for creating a life that accommodates your ADHD and other differences, rather than conforming to standards that do not fit your needs. Clearly, your level of choice and autonomy may be more or less depending on the level of marginalization or privilege you hold with the normative systems which exist in western, capitalist societies.

Self-understanding: Coaches help you uncover how your unique brain wiring operates, fostering deep personal insight that is crucial for effective self-management and personal growth.

Empowerment: Coaching encourages you to view your ADHD difference as something which can be supported and empowered by tasks and environments as well as a strengths-based approach. This shift from an internalized deficit-focused view to a more discerning perspective allows you to leverage your strengths while addressing your challenges in a supportive context.

Navigating barriers: ADHD coaching involves identifying and developing strategies to overcome the societal and practical barriers that you face, whether in education, the workplace, or social settings.

Empowering voices and perspectives

By endorsing the social model, this book aims to illustrate that the lived experience of ADHD is not a deficit to be treated but a different way of interacting with the world in relation to the normative that requires understanding and support. 'Nothing about us without us' takes on a powerful meaning here, asserting that those with ADHD must be central to any conversation about them. Further, those with ADHD must be represented fully. By including *all* ADHDers in the ways to meet their needs, we can dismantle stereotypes and advocate for changes that genuinely benefit the ADHD community, such as policy adjustments, educational reforms, and workplace accommodations that respect and utilize the unique abilities of those with ADHD.

By integrating these insights, this book not only challenges the traditional medicalization of ADHD but also highlights how a shift towards a more inclusive and empathetic understanding of ADHD can lead to richer, more effective support systems. We believe coaching should play an integral part in this support system.

WHAT IS ADHD?

We live in a world that predominantly frames ADHD as negative, a disorder, and implies we are somehow broken. It has the words 'deficit' and 'disorder' in the title, but framing your life as 'deficient' is not a great way to begin to understand yourself. In fact, in their 2021 book ADHD 2.0, expert ADHD psychiatrists Dr Edward Hallowell and Dr John Ratey (both fellow ADHDers themselves) suggest a positive reframe of some ADHD traits to

VAST (Variable Attention Stimulus Trait). This is a helpful shift as it provides a way to explore ADHD more positively. We also believe that it describes our experience more accurately. Dr Thomas E. Brown (2017), a clinical psychologist and researcher in the field of ADHD, argues that ADHD affects a broad range of executive functions and should be understood as a developmental impairment of executive functions, not just attention and hyperactivity.

So what exactly is attention stimulus and what are executive functions? How do they help us gain a more nuanced view of ADHD? Let's take a look by breaking these factors down into four key components.

1. Brains wired for 'interest' not 'importance'

ADHDers often exhibit a unique neurological framework in which their brains prioritize tasks based on intrinsic interest rather than external importance (Barkley, 2015). This predisposition means that our motivation is significantly driven by what is immediately stimulating (or interesting), rather than what is conventionally recognized as important. This can lead to difficulties in prioritizing tasks that are crucial (but not necessarily engaging). It can also create challenges in academic, personal, and professional settings where adherence to externally set priorities is required.

So what actually is interest? In the context of ADHD, interest is deeply intertwined with the role of dopamine, a key neurotransmitter in the brain associated with reward, motivation, and attention. Dopamine plays a crucial role in driving the 'interest system' of the brain, which helps to regulate engagement and focus on activities that are perceived as rewarding or fulfilling.

For ADHDers, the dopamine pathways are often less efficient, leading to a need for higher levels of stimulation to achieve the same degree of reward and interest as those without ADHD (Volkow *et al.*, 2009). This understanding is critical because it highlights why traditional methods of motivation, which might work well for neurotypical individuals, can fail to engage those with ADHD. Within more traditional forms of support like therapy or executive/life coaching, this might look like you not managing to follow through on an action committed to during a session and then feeling deep shame or confusion. ADHD coaching keeps this experience of reward and interest at the forefront of the work. In doing so, ADHD coaches prioritize your unique needs and spend more time within a session exploring what these might be and designing post-coaching session actions and what might help get you interested to follow through instead of assuming that you will simply 'do the thing you said you would'. We'll explore this area in greater detail in Chapters 3 and 4.

Recognizing the importance of dopamine in sustaining interest explains why ADHDers often seek out highly stimulating or novel experiences and why they might struggle with tasks that others find automatically rewarding, engaging, or simply easier to take action on. These are some examples of this interest that we might bring to coaching:

- **Completing mundane tasks:** For many ADHDers, tasks like paying bills or doing laundry require extreme urgency, deadlines, or other forms of stimulation in order to trigger action.

- **Workplace productivity:** An ADHDer might excel in

high-stress, fast-paced jobs that provide constant novelty, whereas they may struggle with repetitive, monotonous roles.

- **Academic challenges:** ADHD students often engage more with subjects they find inherently interesting or hands-on, while they may struggle or avoid subjects that fail to stimulate their brain.

- **Social interactions:** Engaging in conversations with novel or stimulating topics can hold an ADHDer's interest, but something like managing finances with a partner or making polite conversation might be challenging and lead to disengagement.

- **Exercise habits:** ADHDers may prefer high-intensity, adrenaline-pumping activities rather than slower, more gentle activities as the former better sustains their interest and motivation.

This understanding is not only critical for us to understand ourselves but also for educators, employers, and anyone involved in our support system. It highlights the importance of creating environments and tasks that align with our unique needs for stimulation. By recognizing and accommodating these needs through an ADHD coaching relationship, we can design strategies that harness our strengths rather than trying to force us into inherently challenging conventional moulds.

It's helpful to understand that we generate interest (not often consciously) in multiple ways:

- **Anxiety/Fear:** Interest can be sparked by anxiety or fear; the wish to avoid negative outcomes or confront challenges captures our attention. This type of interest motivates actions to mitigate risks or solve problems that provoke anxiety. Over time, relying on this high-stakes motivator can lead to what is termed 'survivor mode' and we will explore this experience in Chapter 4.

- **Urgency:** Interest driven by urgency arises when time-sensitive situations demand immediate attention. The pressing nature of these scenarios compels intense focus and swift action, often bypassing less immediate concerns. For instance, we might ignore routine maintenance tasks until a broken pipe creates an urgent need for immediate repairs, showcasing how the critical nature of a situation compels decisive action.

- **Connection with others:** We often excel at forming social connections and have a high need to feel connected with others (Wiener & Daniels, 2016). These social interactions and relationships can also generate interest. For example, we might find sustained interest in a group project or community event due to the collaborative nature and the desire to contribute to a collective goal, highlighting the role of interpersonal connections in sparking interest.

- **Positive interest:** This refers to an intrinsic curiosity or fascination with specific subjects or activities. Natural interest leads to spontaneous and joyful engagement, where the activity itself is rewarding enough to maintain focus and energy. This links to Flow Theory (Csikszentmihalyi, 1975), first defined as a holistic sensation that people have when they act with total involvement. ADHD coach and coach trainer Cameron Gott (2024) distinguished 'flow' from 'hyperfocus' which can occur through negative interest. 'Flow' is a very positive psychological state that typically occurs when a person perceives a balance between the challenges associated with a situation and their ability to meet the demands of the challenge and accomplish the task. The nine elements of flow include challenge-skill balance, action-awareness merging, clear goals, unambiguous feedback, concentration on the task at hand, sense of control, loss of self-consciousness, transformation of time, and an autotelic experience (Beard, 2014; Csikszentmihalyi, 1975). My example of this is going to art class for a set period of time and getting lost in the painting I am doing.

- **Novelty:** Novelty is very interesting and can often be the reason we feel like 'starters' not 'finishers'. For instance, we might become deeply engrossed in a new hobby like photography due to the excitement and discovery sustaining our attention. When the novelty wears off, it can be hard to sustain the interest.

- **Making the important interesting:** Framing importance in terms of personal values can help us to make an important thing interesting. The laundry, for example, might get done as an act of kindness to our partner. The VIA Character Strengths framework (VIA Institute on Character, n.d.).

gives us a language to connect our values to strengths, which can enhance interest. Equally, we can do easy things and become more interested in them by framing them as strengths.

- **Challenge:** We need enough challenge to engage interest. If it feels too easy, we will disengage.

2. Now versus not now: The ADHD perception of time

Our perception of time, characterized by the 'now' versus 'not now' dichotomy, profoundly affects how interest is generated and sustained (Brown, 2017). We often experience time in extremes: something needs to be done immediately ('now') or it feels infinitely postponable ('not now'). This somewhat binary view of time directly influences motivation and engagement with tasks. For instance, a task may only capture interest when it becomes urgent, thus transitioning from 'not now' to 'now'. This urgency then triggers a rush of interest, primarily driven by the immediate need to address or complete the task before consequences set in (Barkley, 2015).

It's sometimes said that we experience 'time blindness', but this term is unhelpful because it suggests a deficit in our perception of time against a normative ideal. Instead, it's more accurate to describe our experience as 'time perception differences'. These differences can indeed pose challenges in managing procrastination and effective time management, as tasks without interest (such as immediate deadlines) fail to prompt action. However, these differences can also be beneficial. We are often excellent at responding immediately to situations, showing an impressive capacity for rapid decision-making and action in urgent scenarios.

> I was recently refused an emergency exit seat by an airline because I was wearing the Hidden Disability Sunflower Lanyard. The assumption made by the airline was that I could not be relied on in a crisis to assist cabin crew exit because of my 'disability'. The irony is that my ADHD means that I am exactly who you want to be sitting in the exit row in the event of a crisis.
>
> **ALEX CAMPBELL**

Similarly, Katie met someone at a business event who told her he had discovered his ADHD after a very successful ten years in the British Army. His interest in managing crisis situations made him an excellent officer. He described it as 'lucky' that he only found out after he had left because he would not have been allowed to join the Army if they had known.

This adaptability and responsiveness can be a significant strength in dynamic environments, highlighting the value of understanding and leveraging these unique time perception differences. This mechanism underscores the intricate link between how we perceive time and how we engage with tasks based on our level of interest. Within an ADHD coaching conversation, these differences can be unpacked so that you can learn to develop your own strategies that align with your unique ways of processing and engaging with time.

3. Executive functions: The brain's management system

Executive functions are essential brain processes located primarily in the prefrontal cortex, just behind your forehead. They help regulate thoughts, emotions, and actions, allowing us to plan, focus, remember instructions, and manage multiple tasks. For ADHDers, the concept of interest is crucial, acting like fuel that powers these powerful cognitive processes and enhances the ability to manage daily activities.

Research shows that executive functions can be impaired by up to 30% compared to neurotypical individuals (Barkley, 2015). Neuroimaging studies using functional MRI (fMRI) have revealed both structural and functional differences in the ADHD brain. These studies show that while there may be structural differences, such as smaller brain volumes or variations in the prefrontal cortex, the more significant effects are seen in how these brain areas operate and communicate (Shaw *et al.*, 2007). Specifically, pathways related to executive functions, attention, and self-regulation show reduced activity or atypical activation patterns compared to neurotypical individuals.

These functional differences affect the activity of key neurotransmitters, such as dopamine and norepinephrine, which are crucial for regulating attention and executive processes (Arnsten, 2009).

We find that Brown's (2017) Executive Function model helpfully highlights six clusters of our executive functions:

- **Activation:** You may have varying levels of engagement when organizing tasks, setting priorities, and starting projects, often influenced by how meaningful or stimulating the tasks are perceived to be.

- **Focus:** Attention management varies, with differences in maintaining, shifting, and focusing attention based on the task's interest and relevance.

- **Effort:** The regulation of alertness and sustaining effort can fluctuate, influenced by intrinsic motivation and the perceived reward from the activity. Processing speed also varies based on current cognitive and emotional states.

- **Emotion:** Emotional responses can be more intense, with heightened sensitivity to emotional stimuli, affecting how emotions are regulated and moderated.

- **Memory:** Working memory, which is the ability to temporarily hold and recall information, can vary significantly depending on the task's context and engagement.

- **Action:** Monitoring and self-regulating actions can differ, requiring environments and tasks that align with personal management strategies to optimize effectiveness.

Understanding these differences in executive functions can help you develop strategies to manage the ways in which you process and engage with tasks.

Sonny Jane Wise (2024) proposes viewing these executive function challenges as *differences* rather than *deficits*. The extent to which these differences are perceived as strengths or challenges depends on the task, individual interest in it, the sensory environment, and the social context, as well as the individual's physical and emotional state at the time. For instance, our ability to edit this book can vary significantly based on whether we are well rested, fed, and energized, or tired, hungry, and frustrated!

A	Activation	Organising, prioritising & activating on tasks
F	Focus	Focusing, sustaining attention & shifting focus
E	Effort	Regulating alertness, sustaining effort & processing speed
E	Emotion	Managing frustration, regulating & modulating emotions
M	Memory	Utilising working memory & accessing recall
A	Action monitoring	Action monitoring, self-regulating behaviour & pace

Figure 1.1: Executive Functions model

Source: Adapted from Dr Thomas E. Brown's Executive Function model (2005). © 2024 by Gold Mind Academy.

4. ADHD and sensory differences

Understanding ADHD from the perspective of sensory differences offers a crucial lens through which to view the variability in how we interact with our environments. Sensory processing challenges, although not universally present in all individuals with ADHD, can significantly affect their experiences and behaviours. This may also depend on our overlapping traits and co-occurrences with autism, dyslexia, dyspraxia, Tourette's, bi polar disorder, and so on.

Sensory sensitivity in ADHD can involve heightened responsiveness (hyper-sensitivity) or less responsiveness (hypo-sensitivity) to environmental stimuli such as sounds, lights, smells, or tactile sensations, which can be either underwhelming or overwhelming. For some, this might manifest as a distracting irritation caused by the hum of fluorescent lighting or the texture of clothing, while for others, it might be a lack of response to typical sensory input (Yochman, Parush, & Ornoy, 2004). These sensory differences can lead to difficulties in regulating engagement and attention to tasks, particularly when environments are over- or understimulating.

External stimuli

The ability to manage external stimuli plays a significant role in the daily functioning of ADHDers. External sensory inputs like noise, light, and touch can either heighten awareness or lead to overstimulation. Adjustments in the environment can be made to accommodate these differences, such as:

- reducing background noise with noise-cancelling headphones
- using softer lighting to minimize glare and discomfort
- incorporating tactile fidget toys to help manage sensory needs.

Here Alex gives an example of how the external stimuli of sound had a significant impact on his ability to take action (i.e. the executive function of activation) on ordering lunch, even when he knew what he wanted:

I remember a moment with my four-year-old daughter at a busy mall on a Saturday lunchtime. We headed to the food court and I noticed I was feeling unusually agitated, which I initially blamed on my daughter's tantrum. However, when I knew what I wanted to eat but couldn't seem to take action, I became aware of just how overwhelming the noise around me was. Malls, with their glass walls, hard floors, and high ceilings, are terrible for acoustics – sound bounces off every surface, amplifying the chaos. I decided to take us outside, and as soon as we stepped out, I felt my nervous system calming down, and my daughter settled as well. That's when I realized how my brain couldn't filter the sensory overload of sounds, and it was directly impacting my executive function. This insight was a game-changer, and now, I try to avoid malls at peak times.

ALEX CAMPBELL

Internal stimuli

Internal stimuli, including internal bodily sensations and thoughts, can also have a significant impact on us. This includes sensitivity to internal signals such as hunger, pain, or the need to move. Internal sensory processing challenges might manifest as:

- difficulty recognizing internal cues like hunger or fatigue
- a heightened awareness of bodily discomforts or pains
- a need for constant movement or fidgeting to stay focused.

Neuroception

Neuroception, as described by Stephen Porges in his Polyvagal Theory, involves the nervous system's ability to distinguish between safety and threat without conscious awareness. For ADHDers, neuroception can be skewed, leading to heightened states of alertness or anxiety in response to perceived threats (Porges, 2007). This might include:

- reacting to perceived social threats or criticisms (often referred to as rejection sensitivity)
- increased anxiety in unfamiliar or chaotic environments
- difficulty relaxing even in safe situations, due to misinterpreted sensory signals.

The interplay between sensory processing and executive functioning in ADHD can complicate daily activities. An inability to filter out irrelevant sensory data can overload the brain's processing capacity, impairing the ability to focus and execute tasks efficiently (Parush *et al.*, 2007). This sensory overload can lead to behaviours often misinterpreted as typical ADHD symptoms, such as inattention or hyperactivity, but these are instead responses to overwhelming sensory input.

Understanding sensory needs can significantly support executive functioning. Environmental changes, such as reducing background noise or adjusting lighting, along with the use of sensory tools like noise-cancelling headphones or tactile fidget toys, can help regulate sensory overloads. Such accommodations can create a more supportive environment, enhancing the ability to manage tasks and focus effectively.

A spiky profile

A spiky profile refers to a pattern of cognitive strengths and challenges where we exhibit a significant disparity between our abilities and challenges. Common in neurodivergent individuals, it highlights exceptional skills in certain areas, alongside notable challenges in others, contrasting with a more evenly distributed normative cognitive skill set. Nancy Doyle describes it as follows:

> We call this a spiky profile because if you plot their abilities on a graph it will be a big spiky line going up and down. This tells us that neurotypical people are largely generalist thinkers and neurodiverse people are specialist thinkers. (Doyle, 2020)

The challenge here is that in society, and especially in the workplace today, many job roles are designed for that smooth wavy line, not the spiky one. This translates to individuals needing to be all-rounders – quite good at quite a lot of things.

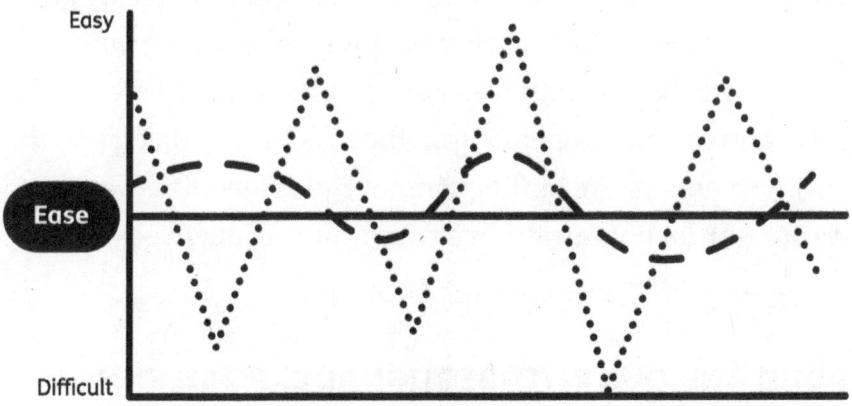

Figure 1.2: Spiky profiles

Source: Adapted from Dr Nancy Doyle's Spiky Profile model (2019). © 2024 by Gold Mind Academy.

Situational variability

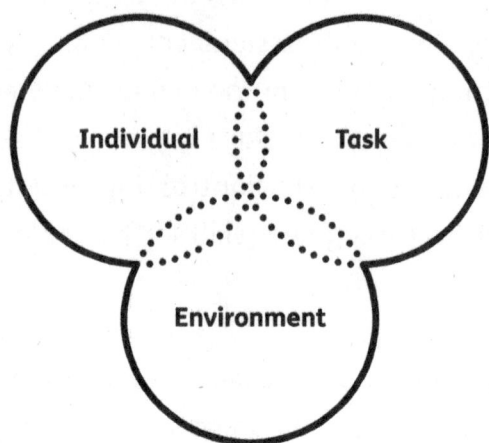

Figure 1.2: Situational variability
Source: Amanda Kirby's TIE model (2021), Do-IT Profiler.

Situational variability refers to the fluctuation in our behaviour, performance, or abilities, depending on the context or environment. This concept recognizes that these variables depend on the Task, Individual, and Environment (TIE) model (Kirby & Smith, 2021), which influences how we function at any given time. If you have a spiky profile and heightened sensitivities – as many neurodivergent thinkers do – you're likely to be very sensitive and variable depending on the tasks you're doing and the environments you're in. 'Environment' also includes the people we are with (or not with!) as well as the time of day/week/month.

ADHD AND OUR INTERSECTIONAL EXPERIENCES

As discussed in the introduction, understanding our ADHD requires a broader social context, recognizing that its medicalization stems from a society that struggles to accommodate differences. The conventional view of ADHD as a purely medical disorder overlooks how societal structures and biases shape the lived experiences of neurodivergent individuals in their multiple identities. These overlapping identities contribute to specific forms of systemic oppression and privilege (Crenshaw, 1989). Just as the feminist movement has historically overlooked the unique struggles of women of colour, Nair, Farah, and Boveda (2024) argue that research on neurodiversity often excludes voices and perspectives from people in the Global South and those racialized and neurodivergent in the Global North. This has the effect of homogenizing neurodiversity into a 'White Neurodiversity Movement', weakening the movement's goals of social justice and equality by not fully representing everyone's experiences.

Similarly, ADHDers are not a homogeneous group and without accounting for the many intersecting differences between us, we are at risk of creating harmful normativity in coaching which can get in the way of the empowerment process that all good coaching, in our view, should facilitate. Normativity protects those with more privilege. This is particularly problematic if the coach holds more privilege and does not acknowledge it in a coaching relationship. Here is an example:

I have a vivid memory of training a group of white male, middle-aged coaches, many of whom had previously worked for a major institution, about neurodiversity. One coach waited until the end of my presentation and pretty much exploded in anger at being presented with what was to him a new idea about difference. He wanted to relate to everyone as 'human', then went on to justify this approach with a recent experience he'd had: a Black woman had asked specifically for a Black female coach and made a sarcastic comment when she came into the room and realized she had been matched with him. He had said, 'Look, let's put aside our differences and get on with what's really important here' and she 'agreed' and according to him they had a 'great' coaching session.

KATIE FRIEDMAN

In this story, the white male coach holds a lot of privilege which they cannot see or actively avoid seeing. This means they cannot see that 'what is really important here' to the client is the intersectional experiences of the client who had spoken up and asked for a specific need only to be completely ignored and the importance of her request, and indeed her identity, negated. What's 'really important here' to the coach is the idea that he can coach anyone and everyone and that this is because he is a really good coach (here by merit). The ways in which the most privileged hide and negate their privilege is discussed in depth by Reeves and Friedman (2024). In this story, the white male coach had interpreted his client's 'going along' with him as him being 'right' and minimizing the importance of difference. It is far more likely that the client no longer felt safe to speak up and had to 'fawn' (a trauma response where someone appeases others to avoid conflict) for her own safety, which may have been something she wanted to explore in more safety with a Black female coach who understood what she was navigating every day.

Sonny Jane Wise, in their 2024 book, *We're All Neurodiverse*, provides a vivid analogy to help us understand intersectionality: imagine standing in the middle of a busy road junction with traffic coming at you from all directions. This situation represents the constant barrage of marginalization and oppression that individuals at the intersection of different identities might face. For instance, as a white, queer, disabled neurodivergent person, Wise experiences privilege from one identity (whiteness), akin to having one empty road at the junction. However, the other roads – queer, disabled, and neurodivergent – bring traffic, representing various forms of challenges and barriers. This analogy highlights how some may face traffic from three directions, while others might confront it from four, affecting their risk and the severity of potential 'hits' or societal challenges they endure.

It is important to add that Crenshaw's term was originally examining the intersection of race, class, and gender and that some intersections will carry more traffic because they are visible rather than the choice of the person to disclose, should they feel safe enough. In an interview for this book, Aisha Thomas describes a resistance to discovering her neurodivergence:

I think the more I began to learn about my son and the more the doctor was asking him questions, the more I realized this was me too!

But in my head, I was thinking, 'I'm already Black. I'm

already a woman. I'm already dyslexic. And now I am supposed to add ADHD or autism or some other label to this
bag I'm already carrying?' So I'm now battling with myself
and I'm thinking 'No, I am not adding that.'

AISHA THOMAS, DIRECTOR OF REPRESENTATION
MATTERS, ADHD-INFORMED COACH

Aisha explores the resistance in the context of other visible intersections and 'traffic' from multiple marginalization, which she
describes as weight she is carrying. She also describes the cost
to her of battling with herself and masking:

What I realized is that the more I was fighting it, the more
it was becoming obvious. It was showing up in my relationships; romantic, platonic, even business. I was becoming
very transactional as it was the only way I could cope: you
do this for me, I do that for you and that's our relationship,
our transaction.

It got to a point where I was putting my friends in boxes:
'My friend for this, does this.' I was compartmentalizing
every aspect of my life, and not realizing that it had anything to do with my brain. I was thinking I was just socially
inept; I didn't have the language or the tools to express how
I was feeling.

A colleague said to me once, 'Your ability to mask scares

me.' You could put me on a stage in front of 2000 people and I would show up and absolutely deliver! Then I could just as simply get off stage and cry. She couldn't understand the switch from what looked like projected happiness to overwhelming sadness. Not because of the work or the subject matter, but instead because I was exhausted from holding it all together.

AISHA THOMAS, DIRECTOR OF REPRESENTATION MATTERS, ADHD-INFORMED COACH

The narrow stereotype of ADHD has also led to underdiagnosis or misdiagnosis of Black and Brown children, whose behaviours are interpreted through the lens of suspicion and scrutiny due to entrenched biases stemming from racial and colonial roots (Coker *et al.*, 2016). As a result, rather than behaviour being interpreted as a need, it is treated with fear, judgement, and control. For example, African American children are more likely to be diagnosed with oppositional defiant disorder (ODD) or conduct disorder, compared to white children who exhibit similar behavioural patterns but are more frequently diagnosed with ADHD (Zulauf-McCurdy, 2023). This can lead to disparities in treatment approaches, with less access to the types of interventions that support ADHD, such as stimulant medications and coaching, and more frequent recommendations for disciplinary actions.

The cost of masking and not fully knowing herself until later in life is clearly shown in Aisha's experience as a Black, multiply neurodivergent woman. Applying an intersectional lens to ADHD means acknowledging that our experiences are profoundly shaped by the environments and systems we are navigating and the safety we experience. The extent to which we mask, and the energy masking takes, is linked to how compromised our safety may be due to the extent to which we are privileged or marginalized.

Historically, ADHD was perceived as a 'disorder' primarily affecting young, white, economically privileged boys whose outwardly disruptive and hyperactive behaviour afforded curiosity and further explanation rather than just punishment and judgement or dismissal. We can see this in Alex's story, a cis white, privately educated male diagnosed with ADHD at the age of four. However, we also learn from his story that the privilege of finding out and accessing support early was not straightforward in the 1990s. There is also a privilege in being an adult who chooses to acknowledge their differences rather than a child who is given a label often to rationalize what is perceived 'wrong' with them.

Cis-women and those gendered as female from birth with ADHD are more likely to exhibit less overt symptoms such as inattentiveness, internalized hyperactivity, anxiety, and depression, which can be mistaken for mood disorders or be overlooked entirely (Quinn, 2005). The lack of recognition of how ADHD presents in girls and women, and those gendered as girls and women, leads to many reaching adulthood without a diagnosis, contributing to ongoing struggles in their personal, academic, and professional lives. If we add the social model to these 'less overt symptoms' we can understand this as a process of socialization. Societal expectations often dictate that women should be more compliant, organized, and emotionally regulated, which can lead to them masking their ADHD symptoms and experiencing internalized distress and self-blame.

Pippa describes how her socialization into a normative 'good girl' and 'helpful girl' got in the way of accessing support for her ADHD, and the cost this had on her time and energy:

ADHD was not a term I'd ever come across, and I just thought I wasn't very bright, that I was 'less' and needed to 'try harder', 'do more'. I wanted to fit in, meet expectations, and fly under the radar, because 'good girls' do not make a fuss. Being cooperative and compliant seemed to be what was required by my parents and my teachers; this was what got me the 'positive feedback', so that is what I learned to do. I got recognized for kindness and being helpful, so I embraced that, being the 'best' friend I could be, the most 'helpful' member of the school community. No one saw my potential; there was no expectation that I would continue in my education beyond 16.

With hindsight I can see my socialization as a girl, the gender bias I experienced, and how my desperate need to fit in fed into that narrative as a 'perfect storm', adding fuel to my internal dialogue of self-limiting beliefs.

I did make it to university. The truth is that I taught myself to overcompensate and 'over learn', and I had to work twice as long for half as much – but I never appreciated that it was due to a neurological difference. I just thought I had 'scraped in' and was not really 'up to it'.

I told myself I had 'high standards' but the reality was that I lived in a state of hypervigilance, just waiting for the next 'snaffu' to bite me on the bum! I had a deep sense that other women were in receipt of the 'secret of managing', and that I clearly had missed it! I needed external validation, recognition, and praise to feel good about myself, but whatever I received, it was never enough. I kept pushing myself. I think I presented as 'busy' but 'on top of it' – but no one saw the cost to my time and energy.

PIPPA SIMOU, CHARTERED COACHING PSYCHOLOGIST AND ADHD-INFORMED COACH

In Pippa's account of her education, we can see low expectations, compliance, minimizing achievements, overcompensating, and a huge amount of effort to keep up when unsupported. One might think that there was little hope of getting a diagnosis given the limited knowledge of ADHD 'back then'.

However, these stereotypes of women are still barriers to getting access to diagnosis in the workplace. Here, Nikki Hardy explains how her differences were explained through stereotypes about her dietary choices rather than her brain wiring:

What did they see, a 43-year-old woman who was a popular staff member, funny, sensitive, caring, a vegan – this is something that so many people put my 'differences' down to – being a vegan! Everything else was disregarded.

Looking back, clear indicators were present. Chronic lateness, cluttered workspaces, my desk was piled high with mess, although this was a huge benefit when hot desking was introduced because no one would want to sit at my desk. Always behind with my paperwork, neglected expenses, recurring absences with depression and anxiety – this should have raised concerns, especially within the clinical setting where I worked and where you would hope clinicians would be attuned to those challenges.

I'm convinced that if I hadn't stumbled on that article and the link to the test, I'd still be in the same place, with all the signs of ADHD being dismissed and overlooked. I'd continue to be labelled as simply a quirky, scatterbrained, funny, disorganized, vegan woman, with occasional bouts of depression – which I now recognize as burnout. Both before and after my diagnosis, this perception persisted, and I've lost count of the number of people who doubted the validity of my diagnosis.

NIKKI HARDY, ADHD CAREER COACH

The experiences of Aisha, Pippa, and Nikki exemplify how intersecting marginalization impacts the acceptance, recognition, and understanding an individual is afforded by normative society. The contributions highlight how norms, biases, and differing expectations can mask or minimize ADHD symptoms and understanding, leading to delayed or missed recognition and support. Understanding these intersectional experiences is crucial for developing a more equitable and tailored approach to ADHD support. While intersectional marginalization causes multi-layered trauma, having space to understand this complexity in order to gain clarity can be very healing.

TRAUMA AND ADHD

Trauma (derived from the Greek word for 'wound') can affect us all differently. It's important to start with the fact that ADHD is not inherently traumatic; rather, trauma arises from a lack of understanding and support in our environments. For ADHDers, trauma often results from negative experiences over time, both during childhood and as an adult. These adverse experiences are exacerbated by living in a world not designed with neurodivergent individuals in mind. Trauma usually stems from not having needs met and/or challenges supported.

It is helpful to frame trauma within two categories: 'small t' and 'big T' trauma (Briere & Scott, 2014; Shapiro, 2001). 'Small t' traumas are personal experiences that, while not life threatening, have a significant and lasting emotional impact, such as chronic criticism, discrimination, or exclusion. For instance, studies show that children with ADHD are often subjected to significantly more criticism than their peers, which can contribute to internalized negativity and self-stigma (Faraone et al., 2015). A child with ADHD will have received about 20,000 times (about 80%) more criticism than the average child for behaviours that they don't understand or do intentionally (Dodson, 2016). This leads to the internalization of negativity which we feel as internal wounds; like thousands of paper cuts which – if there is no healing over time – become open wounds.

This constant criticism, a form of 'small t' trauma, can compound over time, leading to severe emotional distress, ongoing stress, and pain. If these experiences are not addressed, they can contribute to 'big T' trauma, manifesting as severe anxiety or depression later in life. This dynamic illustrates the critical need for supportive environments that understand and cater to the unique needs of ADHDers.

When we consider the ADHDer through their intersectional identity in the context of trauma, the hits of oncoming traffic, and the energy it takes to try and swerve the traffic, cause trauma wounds: sensitivity, traumatized nervous systems, and chronic disease and fatigue. The continual oncoming traffic can be understood as 'small t' trauma, which, over time, leads to 'big T' trauma – or paper cuts, which over decades have become big wounds that we may or may not be treating. Individuals with less intersectional privilege may face more frequent and severe trauma, compounded by limited access to resources for healing (Friedman & Sterling, 2019).

Angela Barnes, a British comedian diagnosed with ADHD after being on antidepressants for 20 years, makes the distinction between ADHD and the traumatizing experience of not understanding herself: 'ADHD was never the problem, not knowing was' (2022).

Our differences are not inherently bad; they are simply different. However, trying to fit into normative systems (which privilege white, male, heterosexual, cis-gendered, able-bodied neurotypicals) leads to internalizing the belief that our differences are flaws, causing trauma as we feel fundamentally 'wrong'.

Inner world of not knowing model

When individuals are receiving negative messaging about their differences which they themselves do not fully understand, it can manifest in three common, unhelpful ways:

Thought: 'I don't want to feel like this.'

Action: Engaging in destructive behaviours such as drinking, drug taking, or risky activities to numb ourselves.

Thought: 'I just need to do better, be better, and try harder.'

Action: Overworking, leading to inevitable burnout.

Thought: 'Everyone else is just better than me.'

Action: Discounting and not understanding or believing in any strengths or abilities.

Recognizing these patterns is crucial to breaking the cycle of self-destructive behaviours and moving towards healing and understanding.

We often experience co-occurring mental health conditions such as anxiety, depression, and substance abuse disorders. These co-occurrences are frequently exacerbated by the challenges and frustrations of living with undiagnosed or unsupported ADHD. Anxiety and depression, for instance, can stem from repeated failures and struggles in academia, work, or social settings, where individuals feel misunderstood or unable to meet expected norms (Barkley, 2006).

The chronic stress of trying to cope with undiagnosed ADHD can lead to significant emotional exhaustion and mental health issues. Additionally, experiences such as substance abuse, self-harm, and disordered eating can emerge as coping mechanisms for the emotional pain associated with these repeated negative experiences and self-esteem issues. The compounded effect of these challenges can create a cycle of mental health struggles that are both a result of, and contributors to, the difficulties of living with unknown ADHD and neurodivergence.

Here, Allie Warren talks about her experience of not under-standing herself, her coping mechanisms, and the impact not knowing has had on her mental health:

Struggling with my mental health has been something that has followed me throughout my life. Without any other diag-nosis, I felt so lost because I was repeatedly told that I was 'just' depressed, but no amount of medication or therapy seemed to help. I spent decades feeling like such a failure and that it must be my fault that I couldn't manage life in the same way that other people seemed to.

Throughout my twenties, I used alcohol to mask how uncomfortable I was in social situations, often to excess and on many occasions, put myself in risky or even dangerous situations. I didn't know how to feel comfortable in my own skin, and constantly looked to others for validation.

I always found it really difficult to know what to do in social situations with friends and at work. Sometimes I would be told that I was too much and over the top, so I would try to be less and then would be told that I was too quiet or too boring. I was so desperate to belong that I started to simply mirror what other people were doing in the hope that this would help me to be the person that I was 'supposed' to be, until I had no idea who I was any more.

In my working life, I spent decades trying to find something that 'fitted' who I was supposed to be. I would start something new and it would become my whole focus; I would feel inspired and excited to learn new things before becoming bored and depressed, and so the cycle repeated itself.

And everything just felt really hard, all the time.

ALLIE WARREN, ADHD COACH AND WORKPLACE CONSULTANT

As well as trauma over time, we can experience 'big T' trauma due to our neurodivergent traits. Literature suggests that ADHDers are more susceptible to impulsivity and engaging in risk-taking behaviours, and have difficulty in foreseeing the consequences of their actions (Hinshaw, 2018). This heightened exposure to risky situations can lead to a vulnerability to more frequent traumatic experiences. Allie mentions risky situations and the reliance on alcohol as a way of coping and creating certainty. ADHD can make us more socially naive, and more likely to find ourselves in situations we later regret.

However, by labelling our experiences in the context of trauma within supported spaces, we can learn how our wounds present in our bodies and how to thrive while carrying and healing these wounds.

The ADHD fight song of accessing help once you have found out

For many ADHDers, the experience of 'finding out' involves accessing help from normative systems which can cause further trauma and exhaustion. Here, Nikki describes her experience of navigating resistance to getting her needs met in the workplace:

In my capacity as an employment specialist, my primary responsibility involved helping individuals in their return to employment or in retaining their current positions. Sadly, I encountered unexpected resistance from my manager. This was in stark contrast to the support I had provided to others in similar situations, highlighting the complexities that can arise when advocating for one's own needs.

I was clear on what I needed to help me: ADHD coaching from someone with lived experience, Dragon software, a dictaphone, and noise-cancelling headphones. I understood how crucial these tools would be in my ability to undertake my role. Despite securing funding for ADHD coaching through Access to Work, I was advised to undergo counselling through the Employers Assistance Programme, which

I knew was not what I currently needed, having already sought counselling years before my diagnosis.

I was asked to write a business case for why I needed ADHD coaching. Having to justify my need, particularly from someone with lived experience, felt unjust. My manager didn't see the lived experience part as necessary, which added to the frustration. Moreover, being required to outline how this support would benefit the service and KPIs in a business case felt outrageous. It seemed like an unnecessary hurdle in accessing the support I knew would greatly assist me in my role.

Below is the last section of my business case. The part where I mention that it will make me a more effective, efficient employee makes my blood boil now:

> 'I feel with the above recommendations, it will allow me to be able to progress further, be more productive, manage my time more efficiently, help greatly with my well-being and confidence, and make me a more effective and efficient employee.'

I was pressured into this.

ANONYMOUS

Burnout is a significant risk for ADHDers, often precipitated by continuous efforts to cope with their undiagnosed neurodivergent needs in environments structured around neurotypical expectations. Many adults report discovering their ADHD following a burnout episode, having endured multiple burnouts throughout their lives. This repeated cycle of burnout can lead to a crucial realization about the role of ADHD in these patterns, highlighting the importance of understanding one's neurodivergence and addressing unique needs proactively (Friedman & Sterling, 2019).

Those of us navigating more intersectional identities that do not fit norms that systems are built for will enjoy less autonomy, choice, clarity, and safety. For example, for menopausal women, their safety in work or in the medical system is already compromised due to work policies and medicine that centre the white male experience. Criado Perez (2019) states, 'The result of this deeply male-dominated culture is that the male experience, the male perspective, has come to be seen as universal, while the female experience – that of half the global population, after all – is seen as, well, niche.' If we add the general misunderstanding of neurodivergence and its situational variability to the already jeopardized understanding of a menopausal woman, the lack of understanding and safety is likely to have a compounded toll on our nervous system and, consequently, our bodies.

Elaine describes how the medical system missed and dismissed her symptoms, and the personal research, persistence, and economic privilege it took to get effective healthcare:

By 2014, I had taken extended time off work on three separate occasions due to 'stress'. Thanks to private healthcare, I accessed a psychiatrist quickly and was diagnosed with depression, anxiety, and obsessive compulsive disorder (OCD).

In 2018, as my mental health declined again, I started hearing about women being misdiagnosed with mental health conditions when their symptoms were actually related to peri/menopause. Armed with this knowledge, I visited my psychiatrist, convinced that my symptoms were menopause-related – after all, I had almost every symptom on the 'menopause bingo card'. Yet, each time I mentioned it, clinicians dismissed my concerns.

I couldn't understand why tasks like retaining information, researching, and writing reports had become so difficult when I had once managed large projects with ease. In desperation, I decided to take an online ADHD questionnaire. The results indicated a high probability of ADHD. But with NHS wait times stretching up to eight years in some areas, I sought a private diagnosis.

In March 2023, I was diagnosed with combined-type ADHD and began titration onto medication. It took six months to find the right dosage. I'll never forget the first day I took my medication – the quiet in my head, the focus. I felt both elated and cheated, knowing how many years I had suffered unknowingly.

ELAINE TRAVERS, FOUNDER OF TRAVERSE

For Elaine, the years of not knowing and her needs not being met or listened to impacted her mental health, work, and well-being.

When she finally started to seek answers at a point where her symptoms were becoming increasingly severe due to the menopause, she was being underserved by the health system, which is only just starting to talk openly about menopause in general and lacks specialists in ADHD and menopause across the country.

Here is the lived experience of someone who has identified coaching as helping her navigate the complexity of her health needs and advocate for herself in a health system with limited time and knowledge of complexity:

My experience of coaching has helped me disentangle interacting health issues. I realized I also have premenstrual dysphoric disorder (PMDD) and my menstrual cycle has a *huge* impact on my ADHD symptoms. I extensively researched these conditions on my own as it is very rare to get a GP appointment where anyone can talk to you long enough to cover so many interacting health conditions.

I am also learning to adapt to fluctuating energy levels, taking the rest I need when I need it and being kind to myself when my symptoms are bad. I do tell my team when I'm in a low energy week and I might need them to help me out more than normal. They are incredibly supportive.

I have also discovered a lot of trauma in coaching that I started to realize I would need therapy for and I have pushed for an NHS referral. I have self-referred to this service before, but because I wasn't experiencing depression or anxiety, I was told they could not help me. This time, I was finally able to articulate my symptoms effectively and secure a six-week course of therapy (Eye Movement Desensitization and Reprocessing, EMDR) for depression with active trauma symptoms. I am really looking forward to starting.

ANONYMOUS

The experience of both Elaine and the client above speaks to the complexity of health symptoms, the need to slow down and process experience in order to untangle what is needed, and the importance of being clear regarding your own experience. This is far beyond the time remit a doctor can offer but gaining clarity on needs and considering how to access further support is a function of ADHD coaching and supports precision healthcare.

Many ADHDers talk about an initial euphoria in finding out and going into a hyperfocus to learn about their brains and then what can be a real low when realizing they still find things hard and some things can't change. For those of us having to rely on over-stretched state-funded support, we may have lost all hope in accessing support at all:

You do start – in my experience of diagnosis – not much better off. For me, it was probably worse for years because specific clinics within the NHS – where I accessed my first ADHD support – just couldn't physically supply helpful support. In these surroundings of information there's bandwagons and miracle cures for everything – and even more importantly money to be made from it. So the well-meaning systems become stretched to non-existence. It's like the wolf cleverly appearing as grandma – the irony is both scary and hilarious.

The scary part is that you give up, you accept the wolf for the wolf, and for me this meant going back to a well-trodden path – 'I don't need anyone' and 'they can't help me'. The struggle most certainly got real at this point.

GARETH DAKIN

After (sometimes) decades of being in 'survival mode', ADHDers are very speedy. If you don't – or can't – take the time to pause, understand yourself, and access specialist support, you can end up with very limited knowledge of your ADHD. This, in turn, can take you straight into the spiral of survival narratives as Gareth highlights here:

Knowing you have ADHD doesn't mean you understand it. When you are trained in self-loathing it could be used as an excuse. The storm in the teacup episodes may gain reasoning but the sadness, loneliness, and anger continue to impact the loving support around you just like they've wrecked any support in the past.

GARETH DAKIN

We can inadvertently gaslight ourselves and others by playing down the impact or wondering if we made the whole thing up. Without a nuanced 'behind the scenes' understanding of our ADHD in lots of different scenarios, we might start to see ADHD as a permanent 'problem' rather than highly situational with strengths as well as challenges.

This fixed idea of ADHD as a 'problem' can make us feel powerless and resentful and can lead us to perpetuate negativity and ableism with those around us. We fall into all or nothing thinking and can be taken in by narrow and limiting ADHD stereotypes in order to feel belonging or certainty. Sometimes this presents as humour, and we joke about our ADHD to disarm people and make it feel safer. We might put our ADHD down or stay quiet about it because it remains a source of shame. We can effectively be 'in drama' with our ADHD and ourselves. These are often patterns of survival.

THE DRAMA OF SURVIVAL

Throughout this chapter, we have delved into the complexities of ADHD, revealing that ADHD brains are wired for interest rather than importance. We've explored the differences between the medical model, which focuses on deficits, and the social model, which highlights societal barriers. We've also examined our intersectional identities and co-occurrences, acknowledging that without a comprehensive understanding of these factors, we can find ourselves in a state of confusion and self-doubt. This cumulative experience is what we term 'survival mode' – a state that ADHD coaching aims to transcend by creating certainty, clarity, and eventually choice, helping you to thrive rather than merely survive.

Survival mode is a reactive state where one operates based on immediate needs and stress responses, often characterized by feelings of overwhelm, self-criticism, and a sense of perpetual struggle. A helpful framework to unpack survival mode is through Karpman's Drama Triangle (1968).

In the Drama Triangle, survival mode is often characterized by three 'mindset' positions: Persecutor, Victim, and Rescuer. The Persecutor seeks to blame and attack themselves or others, the Victim negates any responsibility or control, and the Rescuer rushes to help everyone else, seeking validation without realizing the exhaustion and resentment of continually spreading themselves too thin or disempowering those around them. If you have been in survival mode without realizing it, you will have numerous ways of normalizing these behaviours.

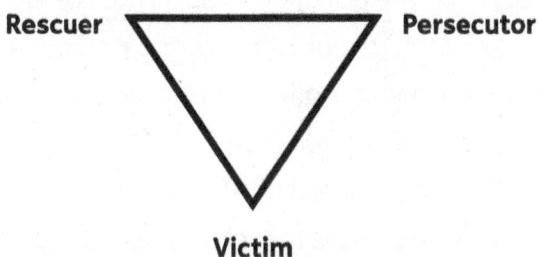

Figure 1.3: The Drama Triangle
Source: Stephen Karpman's Drama Triangle (1968).

My pattern in survival was a tussle between the 'Persecutor' in the form of a vile inner critic, and the 'Rescuer', trying to find solutions by doing whatever it took to try harder and do better. This eventually led me to a spectacular burnout five years ago. I now recognize that this pattern has been continuously prevalent throughout my life, albeit at a lower level. It took me longer to relate to the Victim, but when I started paying attention to my home life, I saw it writ large in my role as a parent who couldn't get kids to do what I wanted in the timeframe I wanted!

KATIE FRIEDMAN

We can see in Katie's example that we may have different survival patterns depending on the situations and environments we are in. If we don't access support and take time to process and understand our differences at a very personal level, we can't disrupt and unlearn the patterns of survival. We end up being in drama with our ADHD/neurodivergence and can't disrupt the 'ableist soup' we have internalized, where messages about being different and disabled are 'less than' or 'bad'.

The danger is that the label of ADHD becomes fixed and negative, and survival responses (which are now decades on in their development of our neural pathways) process the discovery of difference as confirmation of all the reasons there is something wrong with us.

For the Persecutor, ADHD becomes the reason why we are and always have been (insert negative characteristic or story). For the Victim, ADHD becomes the reason there is no point, the reason why we can't and are powerless. For the Rescuer, ADHD becomes an incessant search for tools and tips to fix them.

We have so far looked at the Drama Triangle from an ADHD perspective of survival and as a consequence of 'not knowing'. Unfortunately, there is also a neurobiological lure to the Drama Triangle which is more significant for neurodivergent thinkers. All brains have a negativity bias, an evolutionary feature designed to help us survive (Dethmer, Chapman, & Klemp, 2015), but if ADHDers are wired for interest, then negativity, drama, and solving the challenge of what is wrong makes negativity even more interesting! We want to keep engaged and stimulated (Hallowell & Ratey, 2021). This is to say, ADHD brains will often fall into thoughts of anxiety and, with their interest-powered brains, they may run away with negative thoughts as these can be extra stimulating.

The purpose of identifying when we are in drama is to raise our awareness and help us to monitor our actions in a way which means we choose how we want to be. However, without knowing what the alternative to drama is, this won't work out well and can induce shame. One of the ways to work towards this is by looking at the opposite of the Drama Triangle: the Winning Triangle.

The Winning Triangle

In contrast to the Drama Triangle, the Winning Triangle provides a framework for positive interactions and self-empowerment. Understanding and applying this model can help you move from survival to thriving, offering a path with more agency and autonomy.

The Coach position (also known as 'Nurturer')

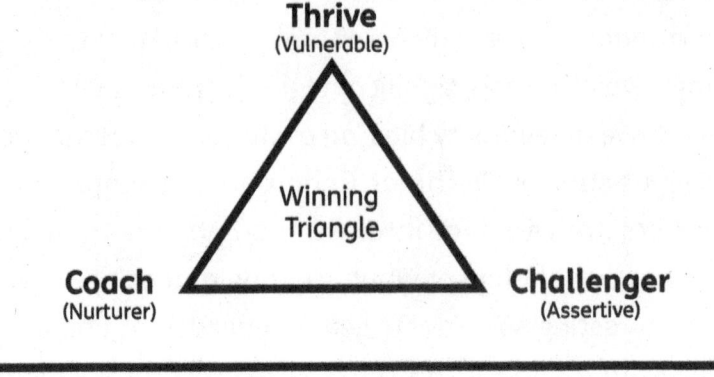

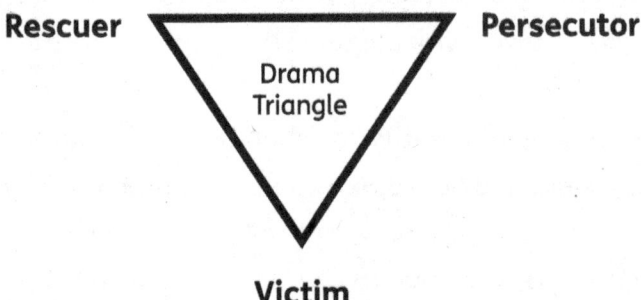

Figure 1.4: The Drama and Winning Triangles

Source: Adapted from Stephen Karpman's Drama Triangle (1968) and David Emerald's Empowerment Dynamic (2005). © 2024 by Gold Mind Academy.

In the Winning Triangle, the Rescuer transforms into the Coach mindset. This position is characterized by curiosity and support without enabling dependency. Instead of rushing to fix problems for others or yourself, you as the Coach ask open-ended questions to encourage exploration and understanding. This means getting curious about our feelings and our reactions rather than suppressing or ignoring them. For example, instead of saying, 'It's fine' when things aren't fine, you might ask, 'Why am I feeling this way? What can I learn from this experience?' This approach fosters self-awareness and promotes proactive problem-solving. It is important to add that if we find ourselves in the Drama Triangle, a winning way to approach this might be to start with 'Coach' and ask what might we be feeling and what might this mean we need rather than persecuting ourselves for being in drama!

The Challenger position (also known as 'Assertive')

The Persecutor in the Drama Triangle shifts to the Challenger mindset in the Winning Triangle. This position involves setting boundaries and speaking up for yourself in a constructive manner. For many ADHDers, embracing the Challenger role can be difficult because it feels confrontational or unfamiliar or we fear rejection for speaking up. However, it is essential for personal growth, maintaining healthy relationships, and protecting our ability to thrive. The Challenger's intention is to invite change and growth, not to harm or judge. It involves articulating needs and expectations clearly and assertively; for example, 'I need more time to process this information' or, 'I feel overwhelmed by these tasks; can we prioritize them together?' This position can need a lot of practice, and a good ADHD coach will be able to help you explore this role in different situations.

The Thrive position (also known as 'Vulnerable')

The Victim transforms into the Thrive mindset in the Winning Triangle. Thriving involves recognizing your needs and actively seeking ways to meet them, rather than waiting for a rescue. This position is about leading with vulnerability (Brown, 2018) and taking responsibility for your own well-being. For ADHDers, thriving might involve identifying specific supports needed to succeed and then pursuing them, such as saying, 'In order to thrive, I need regular check-ins with my manager' or, 'I need to have less going on at the weekend so that I don't become dysregulated.' Thrive means taking charge of your life and making intentional choices to enhance well-being and success. Thrive means getting curious about what works and doesn't work for you and reflecting on what might need to change or be adapted. It is the opposite of pretending we are fine when we are not. Thrive can look like being really honest with ourselves when we are not 'thriving', and seeking support to thrive in the longer term.

The goal here is not to simply be in the Winning Triangle more often. It's about increasing our awareness of when we are in the Drama Triangle so that we can open up possibilities for choice and change. Recognizing our patterns and consciously choosing to adopt the roles of Coach, Challenger, or Thrive can lead to more fulfilling and less reactive lives.

Understanding the Drama and Winning Triangles offers a powerful framework for managing ADHD. By recognizing and shifting from survival mode to a winning mindset, we can break free from the cycle of negative behaviours and build healthier, more effective strategies for living. This journey is about continual growth and self-discovery, learning to navigate the complexities of ADHD with clarity, awareness, and empowerment.

Here Anthony Merrick talks about the natural lure to 'Rescuer' in his job as a clinical nurse and how the Drama Triangle helped him to begin to monitor his actions:

Working in health, I have always had a desire to help others to ensure they were happy and supported, often at my own expense – not just at work but within my personal relationships with friends, family, and partners.

We have a tendency to fall into a position of Persecutor, Rescuer, or Victim – not out of a deliberate desire but perhaps out of habit.

If you were to put on our exercise gear, shoes, grab your headphones and head out of the door every day for a run every morning for five years, it is safe to say at some point along the journey this will become a habit.

Brushing your teeth before bed every evening: habit.

Cooking each evening rather than ordering takeout: habit.

Talking down to yourself, supporting others to your own detriment, externalizing blame for your own trouble, all things done for a long enough period: habit.

Deep internalization of these feelings and behaviours, building them into your personality or day-to-day procedures will make them a part of you as much as going for a run each day or brushing your teeth.

The Drama and Winning Triangles encourage us to break these cycles, shifting this deep internalization of feelings and behaviours and working to alter them if we are willing to make changes.

This internalization, however, is often not just your own actions but the perspective of others and society at large. The expectation of society is that as a professional nurse you take on the troubles of others. When I introduce myself as a nurse I face these expectations, whether they be self-sacrificing my time or my physical and psychological health.

Coaching has allowed me to realize that I can work within a framework, both as a nurse and as a person, that doesn't have to fall in line with societal expectations. I can assertively express myself about expectations within work and push back on perspectives that are not within my responsibility. This process allows me to shift to a more empowering framework, from Drama into Winning.

ANTHONY MERRICK, CLINICAL NURSE EDUCATOR

In Anthony's account, we can see how his context as a nurse in a hospital environment is encouraging the role of Rescuer. While psychological models are useful, they must also be contextual in application, which is why societal inequities need to be factored in when trying to understand ourselves in coaching. This is because our complex mixture of privilege and marginalization in relation to power structures profoundly affects how we experience our environments. We would suggest that the Drama and Winning Triangles be adapted as shown in Figure 1.5.

Doyle (2020) advocates for a biopsychosocial approach to neurodivergence: 'People are more or less disabled, dependent on the extent of the neurological difference, their history, their demographics and social context.' In the next chapter, we'll take a more in-depth look at how ADHD coaching can empower the shift that Anthony refers to: from drama to winning. We will look at some key elements to ADHD coaching including bringing intersectionality into coaching as part of this biopsychosocial approach.

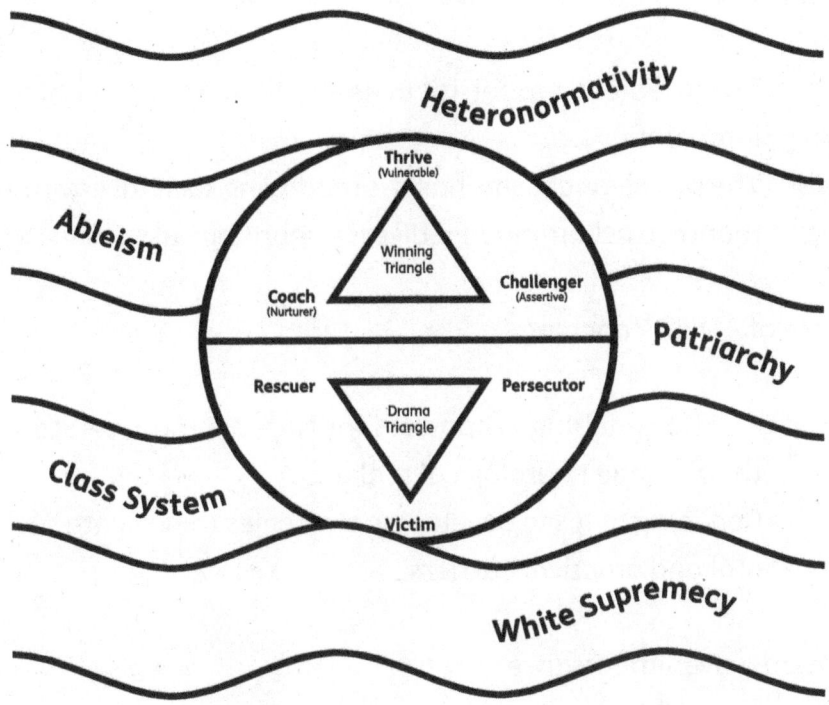

Figure 1.5: Adapted Drama and Winning Triangles

Source: Adapted from Stephen Karpman's Drama Triangle (1968) and David Emerald's Empowerment Dynamic (2005). © 2024 by Gold Mind Academy.

SUMMARY

Key takeaways
Holistic understanding of ADHD:

- ADHD should be viewed beyond the conventional medical

perspective, and recognized for its complexities and the societal barriers that exacerbate challenges.

Medical versus social model of disability:

- The medical model focuses on deficits and clinical interventions.
- The social model emphasizes modifying societal environments to accommodate diverse neurological profiles.

Role of ADHD coaching:

- ADHD coaching empowers individuals to understand their unique neurological makeup.
- Coaching helps in developing strategies to navigate societal and practical barriers.

Interest over importance:

- ADHD brains prioritize tasks based on intrinsic interest rather than external importance.
- Dopamine pathways require higher levels of stimulation for engagement.

Time perception differences:

- ADHDers experience time in a 'now' versus 'not now' dichotomy, affecting motivation and task engagement.
- Understanding these differences helps in developing personalized strategies for effective time management.

Executive functions and sensory differences:

- ADHD impacts various executive functions, which are essential for planning, focus, and managing tasks.
- Sensory processing differences can significantly affect experiences and behaviours, requiring accommodations to manage external and internal stimuli.

Intersectionality and trauma:

- Intersectional identities shape the lived experiences of ADHDers, affecting recognition and support.
- Trauma often results from negative experiences and societal barriers, leading to emotional distress and mental health issues.

Drama and Winning Triangles:

- The Drama Triangle (Persecutor, Victim, Rescuer) represents reactive states in survival mode.
- The Winning Triangle (Coach, Challenger, Thrive) offers a framework for positive interactions and self-empowerment.

REFLECTIVE QUESTIONS

1. In what ways have societal barriers impacted your experience of ADHD?
2. How do you add interest to boring (understimulating)

tasks to help you do them (e.g. listening to a podcast while doing the laundry)?

3. How does your perception of time (now versus not now) affect your ability to manage tasks and deadlines?

4. What accommodations can you implement to manage your sensory processing differences more effectively?

5. How might recognizing your intersectional identities influence the way you seek support for your ADHD?

6. How do you think trauma may have influenced your experience with ADHD and your mental health?

7. Can you identify moments when you have been in the Drama Triangle? How could you shift towards the Winning Triangle in those situations?

8. What steps can you take to move from a survival mode to a thriving mindset in your daily life?

CHAPTER 2

What is ADHD Coaching and How Does it Work?

WHAT IS COACHING?

Before we dive deep into ADHD coaching, it's helpful to understand what coaching actually is and how it differs from other forms of talking support. Here are some definitions:

Mentoring: World Education Services (WES) (n.d.) defines mentoring as: 'a relationship between two people where the individual with more experience, knowledge, and connections is able to pass along what they have learned to a more junior individual within a certain field'.

Therapy (Counselling/Psychotherapy): The American Psychological Association (APA) (n.d.) defines therapy as 'helping people with physical, emotional, and mental health issues improve their sense of well-being, alleviate feelings of distress, and resolve crises'.

Socializing: While there isn't a strict definition for chatting with a friend, it's helpful to recognize what this is so we know how coaching might be different. For the purposes of contrasting, we define this as informal chats characterized by exchanges on common interests, shared experiences, or routine life updates. The emphasis is on maintaining social connections and enjoying each other's company.

Coaching: The International Coaching Federation (ICF) defines coaching as 'partnering in a thought-provoking and creative process that inspires a person to maximize their personal and professional potential. The process of coaching often unlocks previously untapped sources of imagination, productivity and leadership.'

So exactly how does coaching differ from therapy or mentoring? There are four key differences to consider when exploring ADHD coaching:

1. **Focus:** While therapy often focuses on resolving past or present mental health issues, coaching is present and future-oriented, focusing on goal/intention-setting and personal/professional growth. Having said this, while we may not be resolving the past, sometimes the past can be brought in to inform the present and the future. A simple car analogy can help to illuminate this: in order to move forward we may need to check our mirrors and appreciate what is behind us.

2. **Relationship:** Unlike mentoring, which often involves guidance from a more experienced individual, coaching is a partnership between equals where a coach facilitates self-discovery and empowerment without being an 'expert' on you and your ADHD.

3. **Self-directed growth:** Coaching strongly emphasizes self-directed growth. A coach will help facilitate this process, but it is you who sets the goals/intentions and works to achieve them. This is less emphasized in therapy, where a therapist might take a more directive role in supporting you to manage your challenges (depending on the type of therapist). In mentoring, the direction of growth might be influenced significantly by a mentor's experiences and perspectives, and the mentor may hold the mentee accountable.

4. **Client expectations:** Counselling and mentoring often derive substantial value from the insights, awareness, and guidance shared during sessions. In contrast, coaching places a pronounced emphasis on the actions and personal growth that occur between sessions, leveraging the self-awareness and goals/intentions set during sessions to foster transformative changes in your daily life.

It is important to note that while definitions are helpful in making distinctions, coaching borrows and blends from many knowledge domains, including therapy. There are at least 140 different types of therapy and at least the same number of coaching types. Therefore, there is inevitable scope for crossover in both.

WHAT IS ADHD COACHING?

Dolly Parton (n.d.) once said: 'Find out who you are and do it on purpose.' We think this is the essence of ADHD coaching. We are learning who we are to gain certainty and clarity so that we can be us from a place of choice and purpose.

Clearly, 'finding out who you are' is ongoing, intersectional, and complex. Depending on the individual, some of 'finding out who you are' may be or may become the remit of therapy rather than coaching. However, we believe that therapeutic, trauma-informed coaching is most appropriate when working with ADHD, where people have not understood their differences for large parts of their lives.

The Professional Association for ADHD Coaches (PAAC) (n.d.) defines ADHD coaching as 'a specialty skill set that empowers clients to manage their attention, hyperactivity and impulsivity'.

While we agree that ADHD coaching can support you in building skills to better manage your ADHD, we believe its real power lies in something deeper. At its heart, ADHD coaching is about personal development that's rooted in self-awareness and truth. It invites you to explore what thriving actually looks like for you. Not in a generic, one-size-fits-all way, but in a way that reflects your own intersectional context, values, and nervous system. It's about making that felt sense of thriving more accessible, more often, across different parts of your life.

Many of us come to coaching after years spent in survival mode. We may feel disconnected from our feelings, cut off from our bodies, and unsure of what we really need. Jinny Ditzler (2003) paints a helpful picture of this experience by describing three layers of self. You might imagine it like an onion, where the outer layers form over time to protect the tender core. These layers shape how we show up in the world and how unclear we can be on who we really are:

- **Who I pretend to be:** The version of ourselves we present to the world to avoid judgement, fit in, meet expectations, and keep ourselves safer.
- **Who I'm scared I am:** The hidden version of ourselves shaped by shame, fear, internalized criticism, and systemic othering.
- **Who I really am:** The authentic self beneath it all. A complex, whole person made up of situational strengths, challenges, identities, and lived experiences.

ADHD coaching often involves gently peeling back these layers. Coaches offer space to notice and question the masks we wear, the fears we carry, and the deeper truth beneath. It is not about fixing who we are, but about coming home to ourselves with compassion, curiosity, and choice.

This process also happens in the context of larger systems. ADHD coaching includes both personal reflection and a wider systemic lens. It is about returning to who we really are and naming the external forces that have shaped how we see ourselves. When we train coaches, we draw on two sets of competencies to guide this work: one that supports a strong coaching structure, and another that supports trauma-informed, neurodiversity-affirming practice.

ADHD coaching will involve learning to come back to who we really are as well as making systemic challenges explicit. When we train coaches, we adhere to both these two sets of competencies in order to guide the structure of a coaching session:

International Coaching Federation COACHING COMPETENCIES	Professional Association for ADHD Coaches FIVE ESSENTIALS
1. Demonstrates ethical practice	1. Safety
2. Embodies a coaching mindset	2. Collaboration
3. Establishes and maintains an agreement	3. ADHD lens
4. Cultivates trust and safety	4. Wonder
5. Maintains presence	5. Actioning
6. Listens actively	
7. Evokes awareness	
8. Facilitates client growth	

Sources: © International Coaching Federation (2021) & © Professional Association for ADHD Coaches (2020).

As well as supporting the structures above (which are a feature of every session), it is important to visualize the potential trajectory of ADHD coaching so that you can have some much-needed certainty about what to expect and what the 'end' looks like.

It's equally important to underscore that coaching – particularly ADHD coaching – is not about imparting tips and tricks from some 'wise' ADHDer who happens to call themselves a coach. If coaches do not define the potential trajectory and purpose of ADHD coaching, we are likely to ask for advice, tools, tips, and tricks to manage our ADHD.

This is because we have been conditioned to think we need fixing – as well as having a dopamine-driven brain that's looking for quick-fix solutions. Rather than resist or frustrate you, we think painting the bigger picture of ADHD coaching helps you to get interested in the process, connect to your why, and reconfigure expectations with something tangible. This in itself creates safety and collaboration. Knowing how coaching works and what to expect over time can create firm containers for our speedy brains that want to race to the end before they have begun!

In order to aid the understanding of the work that can be done in ADHD coaching, we show this ADHD Needs Pyramid, originally adapted by Robbins' '6 Human Needs' in 2021 from Maslow's Hierarchy of Needs (1943), and which we have adapted further to suit the ADHD discovery journey.

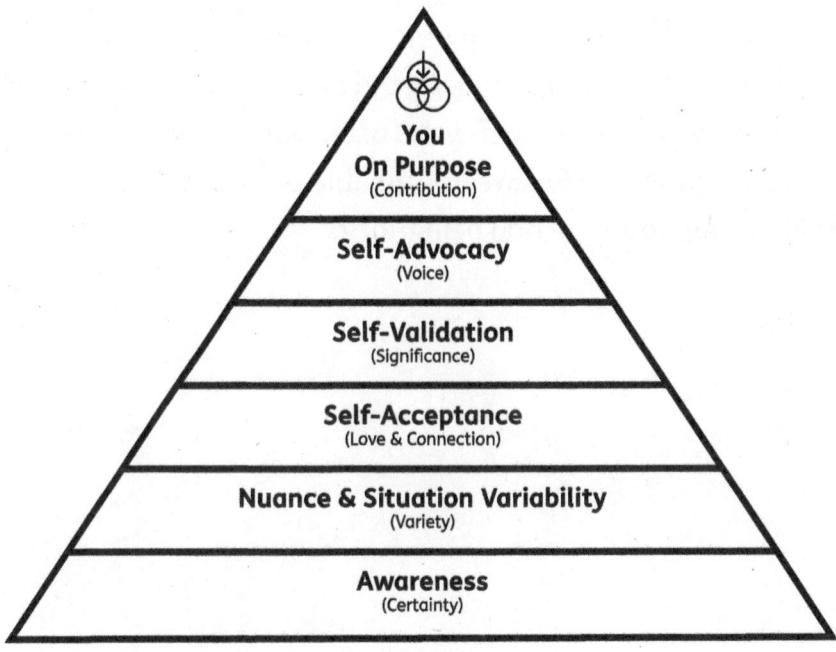

Figure 2.1: The ADHD Needs Pyramid

Source: Adapted from Tony Robbins' 6 Human Needs (2006), based on Abraham Maslow's Hierarchy of Needs (1943). © 2024 by Gold Mind Academy.

Often when we use this pyramid with clients, they reflect on having spent much of their lives trying to contribute without a stable base of certainty. If we have not known who we are and how we are different, the experience can feel more like the inverted pyramid shown in Figure 2.3.

Inevitably, limited certainty and safety regarding how we are different and why will have made our experience of our variability feel like a rollercoaster of ups and downs with no rhyme or reason. This often leads us to doubt ourselves. Love and connection are hampered by not being able to connect with, understand, and rely on ourselves. Without this, we seek validation from others rather than validating ourselves, so other people's opinions become all powerful and rejection can destroy us. Without certainty of our differences, growth can feel like a never-ending endeavour to 'be better' in order to be more 'normal'. Contribution often involves cycles of burnout, or never reaching the contribution we feel we are capable of, or a feeling of never fulfilling our potential and being 'lazy'.

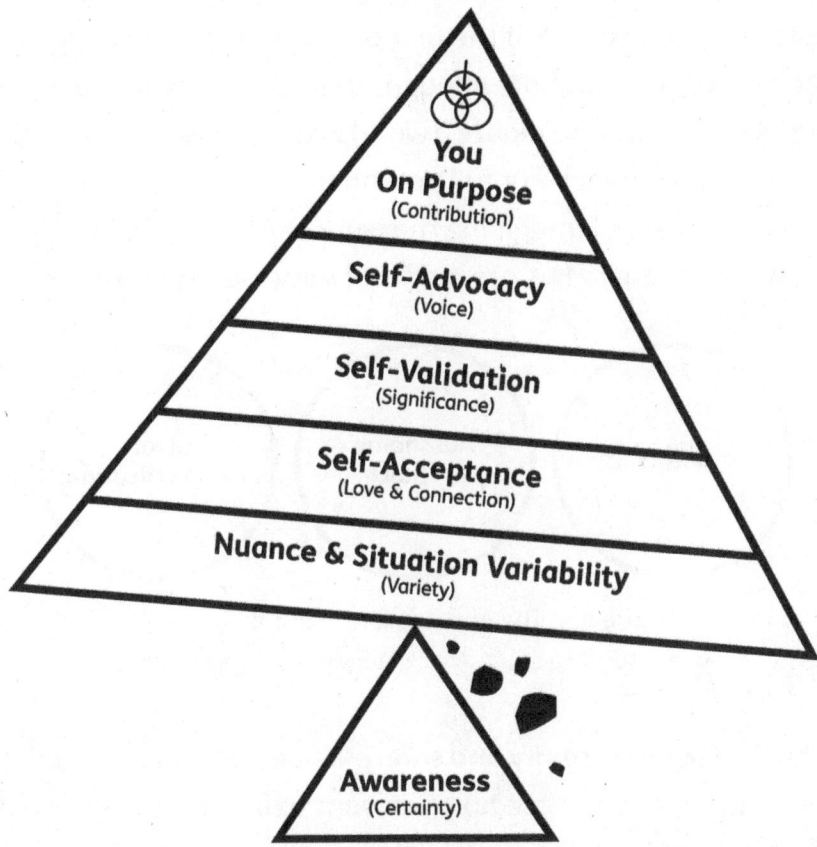

Figure 2.2: The ADHD Needs Wobbly Pyramid

Source: Adapted from Tony Robbins' 6 Human Needs (2006), based on Abraham Maslow's Hierarchy of Needs (1943). © 2024 by Gold Mind Academy.

In ADHD coaching, coaches are aiming to help you build back a wide base of certainty while accommodating and accounting for complex variability. The aim of ADHD coaching is to move away from survival by loving and connecting to ourselves, our emotions, and our needs. ADHD coaching can help us to validate ourselves by starting to see ourselves through our strengths – both when we are thriving and when we are in difficulty. Once this is under way, growth in the form of self-advocacy gets easier because we can let go of the fear of rejection from others (or a need for their validation) enough to speak up and express our truths and we start to realize a world of possibility where we can contribute and reach our full potential.

Another way of imagining the work of ADHD coaching is to use Atif Choudhury (2021)'s model of Anticipatory Inclusion:

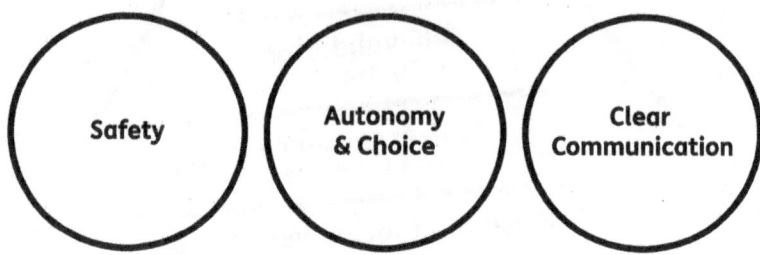

Figure 2.3: The Anticipatory Inclusion model
Source: Atif Choudhury's Anticipatory Inclusion model (2021).

When we build certainty and safety, we become empowered to try things out, to choose how we want to be, and to figure out what we need to support this. Once we have tried and tested what works for us, communication can be much more effective and we can be clear on when it is not where we need it to be from ourselves and others.

The problem with all models is that they imply that change – or indeed the ADHD process – is linear or sequential. In reality, models and visuals are just templates and everyone's process will diverge. The needs described in these models will be governed by what you bring to each session. This could be determined by what you are noticing and reflecting on between one session and the next. It will also come from whatever is happening in your life and what is holding your interest. Visuals and models provide templates of the path ahead but everyone's change process is messy and individual. A client once commented in a final session that they saw their change journey in loops, that they would have never had the confidence to share how they saw it prior to coaching, and that drawing things had been really freeing in finding ways to express themselves.

Regardless of what you bring to each session or how you prefer to process information, there are a number of elements in ADHD coaching which help to bring about change.

Different coach training providers may emphasize different things. We think that it is important to align with the appropriate best practice (such as the ICF and PAAC) while innovating as you go. The key, we feel is to have a clear 'why' for each element:

1. ADHD lens and narrative change.
2. Nuance, intersectionality, and situational variability.
3. Love and connection to ourselves – self-regulation through systematic pausing and emotional granularity.
4. Self-validation through strengths work.
5. Self-advocacy – being assertive as well as nurturing and vulnerable.
6. Putting it all together – you on purpose.

Over the following sections, we'll explore how these tools and core concepts can contribute to your empowerment process.

1. ADHD LENS AND NARRATIVE CHANGE

We usually arrive at coaching with some awareness about ADHD but our knowledge is often received through the medical model which is deficit based and often not personalized to our experience. It's as if we are engaging with ADHD at the theatre and have taken our seats to watch the show, but in reality we need to lift the curtain, go behind the scenes, and become part of the production.

When we are initially spectators, we refer to ADHD as a problem, one which is separate to us. We may try to conform to simplistic ideas around ADHD. At other times we may not see the ADHD in our behaviours and actions and instead interpret them as personal failings or personal strengths that have nothing to do with ADHD.

Here, Lizzie talks about a time where she didn't understand herself in her 'procrastination' and how she manages now that she has the ADHD lens:

I spent the first year of the postgraduate degree that I embarked on in my late forties not knowing that this chaos in my head was my executive function challenges. The challenge with activation was huge. I had no way to describe the fact that I knew what I needed to do, I knew I had a really good brain, I knew that I understood everything, I knew what the deadline was, I knew what needed to be done and yet I would sit for hours and hours and not do any of it.

I had no language for my struggles with activation (that I now know were exacerbated by hormones and Covid) rather than, 'Fucking hell, I'm useless'. And, 'Oh my god, if anybody knew I was up here in this office not doing anything...' I felt so much shame that I could be with my family and I was not working properly up here, but they were trusting that I was.

Since having ADHD coaching, I still find myself doing that but I do it far less. I get out of paralysis faster. I know what it is – 'decision overwhelm', racing to the end and not knowing where to start, and emotional flooding. Now I've also got more options. Instead of just trying to get myself back into it, I might do something else, knowing that I can come back to it.

LIZZIE BENTLEY BOWERS, EXECUTIVE COACH
AND ADHD SPECIALIST COACH

When ADHD is not integrated into our identity, we waste a lot of time and energy, as exemplified here by Lizzie. When we start to work with our brain, we have effectively got out of our theatre seats and got involved in the production of our lives.

In order to accelerate this process and reduce the overwhelm outside coaching sessions, we use visual prompts and frameworks. By learning about our experience and having a series of models (like Brown's Executive Function model, 2013), we start to build memorable hooks that we can hang our experience on. This allows us to access the ADHD lens when we are in difficulty. We frame noticing (including excruciating noticing that we wish we didn't have to notice!) as 'winning' because we can't have choice and agency over what we don't see.

Here Allie talks about having to stop coach training in order to work on her own understanding of herself through ADHD coaching. She describes how hard it can be to notice difficult things without knowing what to do about them:

I remember feeling really frustrated with myself around that time because having to take a break from training felt like failing. Everyone else was fine and managing – why couldn't I do it? But having that time to focus on what I needed and being coached myself has changed my life in every way imaginable.

I understand now that I needed that time to process my autism and ADHD diagnosis and what that meant for me. One of the key elements of coaching is facilitating change, and that change starts with noticing. But with ADHD and autism, a lot of the things that you're noticing can be really difficult. Things like noticing when your emotions are too big and trying to control them is really hard, or noticing that you don't know what emotions you're feeling, so trying to understand how you feel is impossible. Working through those big feelings or feeling shame about some of your behaviours can be really challenging and there's a lot of learning and un-learning on the way.

I've learned how my brain works and why some things are easier and some harder. I've been given a whole new language to understand myself, talk about how I'm feeling, and experiment with ways of being in the world that work for me.

ALLIE WARREN, ADHD COACH AND WORKPLACE CONSULTANT

Allie needed time to process her understanding of her ADHD in the context of her experience and co-occurrence with autism. We often rush into learning experiences because it feels like familiar terrain but when training involves starting with you, we may need more support to get clarity and certainty about who we are in smaller groups or one-to-one settings before we can engage effectively within a bigger group. We often show up differently in different situations and are very sensitive to our environments. The level of safety that anyone feels will be informed by their experiences of marginalization. Understanding how this works for you in your intersectional context is part of tailoring the understanding of ADHD to you.

2. NUANCE, INTERSECTIONAL LENSES, AND SITUATIONAL VARIABILITY

Both Lizzie and Allie talk about the shame and the overwhelm that we hold without this language and understanding and how empowering it is when you have a language to describe your experience. Whenever we try to undo unhelpful shame narratives which have embedded over time, we need to replace them with something more true and often infinitely more positive than the negativity we hold. Before we replace them, we need to get some perspective on where they have come from and how we are encouraged to internalize them. Depending on our intersectionality and the marginalization we experience, the internalization of shame may be stronger. ADHD coaching, like all good coaching, needs to speak to the 'who' of the person (i.e. focusing on the individual's identity and strengths) which may very much be informed by intersectional differences. Unfortunately, mainstream coaching rarely addresses these differences. Here, Minesh talks about the first time his intersectionality was invited into an initial discovery call where coaches establish agreements with potential clients about how they will work together (we discuss discovery calls and contracting in Chapter 3).

My ADHD coach asked me about my intersectional differences and how they might impact my experience in a contracting session. I got stuck and thought 'Wow! I have not had to think about this before and I have never been given the space or the safety to think about this before. I've never felt comfortable or safe enough to really think about it and to share it – to put these thoughts into words.' And I think it is super interesting that I have worked in this bloody space (learning and development) for 20 years and I have been coached so much, I've been line managed by so many people and I have never been asked this. And when my ADHD coach asked this, it brought up a broader perspective of not just having never been asked in coaching but everywhere else where it's important in my life, my family's life, and that of my parents...a question around differences would have been a powerful thing to have... And to be offered to think about differences in that space was powerful and I couldn't put words to it then and I was really emotional and I couldn't figure out why it was so jarring in a good way. I was confronted with, 'Why the fuck was this never asked before?'

If it had been asked in coaching, I would have got to my truth or closer to my truth much quicker. Without that important lens there's code switching, there's masking happening over the real experience. I can't say what the truth is for me because I am worried the coach won't get it because I have not been invited to think about my differences. In the Ditzler model I am staying with who I pretend to be, not even who I am scared I am. I am not willing to face my fear because I am scared of gaslighting by the coach. By not having the conversation, you're not able to hold the multiple traumas but it's there. So I've got this whole load of experience that is just sitting underneath, and asking about ADHD alone won't get to it.

MINESH SIYANI, ADHD SPECIALIST COACH AND
LEARNING AND DEVELOPMENT LEAD

Raising difference and intersectionality may be confronting initially and you may need time to process. If it is invited from the start of a coaching relationship, it can be brought in to evoke awareness and to help you become discerning about the environments you operate in and how they interact with your intersecting identities of marginalization and privilege. Once we can discern our environments, we can get closer to our truth.

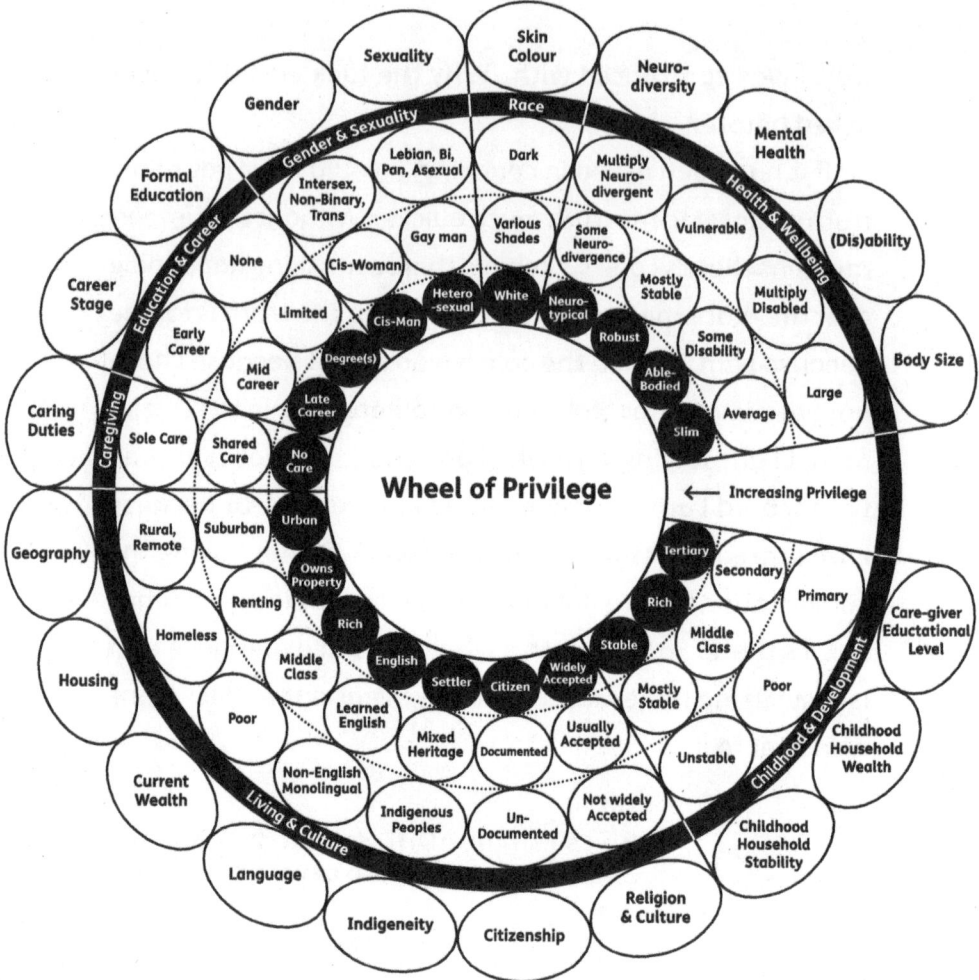

Figure 2.4: The Intersectionality Wheel

Source: Adapted from the Academic Wheel of Privilege (FORRT, 2023), which builds on Sylvia Duckworth's Wheel of Power/Privilege (2020) and the original conception of intersectionality by Kimberlé Crenshaw (1989). Adaptation © 2024 by Gold Mind Academy.

Later, my ADHD coach raised my intersectionality and my differences during a coaching session and she just stayed there and held the space and didn't let her fragility about differences lead her to run away. And then when she brought in the Intersectionality Wheel I really got into it because we had contracted previously and talked about it so when she brought it into a specific situation, it was surprising for me how important that lens was in using the wheel. So if you contract for differences at the beginning you might not get anything but it might lay the trust to bring it in later.

MINESH SIYANI, ADHD SPECIALIST COACH AND
LEARNING AND DEVELOPMENT LEAD

Having experienced the impact of exploring ADHD intersectionality for himself, Minesh uses an intersectional lens to hold space for his clients now that he is an ADHD coach:

Even in a coaching conversation today I acknowledged that we hadn't talked about differences and then the client really shifted her perspective and started to understand her situation at a deeper level: 'Because of my female lens I'm treated like this in retail, because of my Asian lens I feel like I have to say yes to everything, because of seniority and being respectful.' I wouldn't have got that from the ADHD lens alone. So in surfacing difference, it creates more nuance. For example, for me, in saying no in boundaries – there's ADHD and culture and they are different, and just tackling

ADHD doesn't tackle my lens around hierarchy and respect and the issue might be about how to respectfully say no that honours my culture.

In the example above, by understanding situations through our multiple identities, it can help us to understand how we hold some ways of being as important to us and how this informs how we navigate spaces. By gaining clarity on the multiple ways that our identities inform our thoughts and actions, we may find that some of the beliefs come from normative systems that don't serve us. In western capitalist societies, some of us are closer to the norms of white, male, able-bodied, middle-class, heteronormative, cis-gendered privilege than others (to name but a few intersections). By becoming clear on normative systems and how they may or may not be serving us, we are more able to externalize rather than internalize the othering we may experience, and in doing so, create perspective and choice.

It may, at first, feel counterintuitive to acknowledge systemic structures as if this perspective might invite inaction or stuckness. However, if we understand what is easier and more difficult for the ADHD brain (including intersectional ways in which we operate in systems of barriers and privilege), we can start to loosen the internalization of what we have perceived to be 'wrong' with us and instead appreciate what is 'wrong' with society and the messaging it gives us. This helps to ease the shame shutdown and we are often better able to process difficulty, protect ourselves with boundaries, and get clearer in our communication of our needs and how they are different.

The truth will set you free but at first it will piss you off (Gloria Steinem, quoted in Grayson Perry's (2017) book, *The Descent of Man*)

Here Katie talks about a coaching experience where her coach raised the potential power dynamic in her story, which gave her clarity:

I recently had a bad experience when doing a podcast with a male podcaster which, after some useful ADHD coaching, resulted in an assertive conversation and an agreement not to publish the podcast. After going through the nuance in the situation with an ADHD coach and how I was made to feel unsafe through specific actions, my coach also acknowledged that the man was probably intimidated by me because I come across as confident and direct in a way that is unexpected for a woman. Seeing my strengths and appreciating that they intimidate some people is hard for me. By raising it, my coach helped me to appreciate that I do not conform to misogynistic ideas of how women should be and as a result, some men find this more difficult. Rather than feeling stuck or upset by this, I felt empowered to separate what is 'mine' to address and what is 'his' to unlearn.

KATIE FRIEDMAN

Contracting to bring in the ways in which normative systems have impacted you can be very helpful in raising awareness and validating your experience. Many of us are, or have been, masking in order to stay safe, whether we realize it or not. We will all experience different degrees of safety in different environments depending on our lived experience, our intersectional identities, and whether we get to choose our disclosure of these identities or not. In the example above, the coach has made it safe for Katie to acknowledge how patriarchal systems are affecting the people around her and creating expectations that don't work for her. The fact that the coach held male privilege and still acknowledged the system meant a lot to Katie's sense of safety and ability to process in the coaching space.

Here, Lizzie talks about the value of being able to consider ways in which she had been impacted by neuronormative systems and then more broadly about how her other intersectional identities have shaped her experience in ADHD coaching:

The systemic perspective helped me to realize I've got every right to feel the way I feel. And so I think that's probably permission or validation. So instead of it being me versus the world, it was me as part of a group of people who were also part of a bigger group of people. And I think that helps me stay out of some of the less hopeful thinking.

And then through the coaching I was like okay, well what else is at play for me? Yeah, not just ADHD. But perimenopause, early life experiences, and so on.

Once I could account for the system (and me in it), I also realized what was my responsibility and I believed I deserved better. Then things became more possible. I got interested in this because I understood myself. Then it shifted from 'I should do something' to 'I want to do something', and working out how. Discovering one possibility led to another. Celebrating the wins and the strengths really helped with this. I am so grateful to be here rather than where I was. The impact of ADHD coaching was to be able to see myself and my life from somewhere different and better, easier, and kinder. And I remember that I started to realize there were strengths everywhere if you know how to spot them, name them, explore them, develop them. The other thing was hope. ADHD coaching gave me hope back rather than circular judgement and shame internally.

LIZZIE BENTLEY BOWERS, EXECUTIVE COACH
AND ADHD SPECIALIST COACH

The ability of the coach to hold a systemic perspective as well as an appreciation for your intersectional identity is incredibly valuable when facilitating thinking about how the environment and you, the individual, interact in situational variability. If we are able to hold that society is deliberately organized to be racist, misogynist, homophobic, and ableist, we can be discerning about environments and the people in them and how they can be helping or hindering success. We often don't feel safe to be all of us with coaches or therapists, and our sensory sensitivities can make us deeply intuitive to a person's discomfort or fragility. Minesh mentions sensing this fragility in previous coaching experiences. We need ADHD coaches who are willing to work on their own fragility. When asked how he manages his own fragility in coaching, Minesh said:

> It comes where I haven't done the work, the research to orient myself. I don't get it so much with race or gender as I have worked on this but I feel my own fragility around sexual orientation because I haven't done the work. And the key is to notice the fragility, regulate and figure out your feelings, and do the bloody work outside the coaching! Sometimes you have to surface the fragility and commit to action with the client in order to stay present with them – and definitely don't ask them to educate you while paying you!
>
> **MINESH SIYANI, ADHD SPECIALIST COACH AND LEARNING AND DEVELOPMENT LEAD**

We often feel and have more awareness of our marginalization than our privilege. It's likely that the more privilege we hold, the more fragility we will have towards surfacing differences we are not clear about. The key, as Minesh says, is to commit to finding out about differences in order to get clearer. This will serve us in all our relationships. We are more able to truly learn about and understand others when we are clear and connected to our own felt experiences. The way we connect to our bodily sensations and pay attention to our feelings can be influenced by our interoception or the way our body and mind send signals to each other, which can be hyper- or hypo-sensitive in neuro-divergent people. It can also be hugely impacted by environments and systems we have grown up in, as we shall see in the following sections.

While there are many reasons that we may be disconnected from our bodies, as discussed in Chapter 1, one of the first steps for all of us to reconnect to our felt experience is to pause. We can't change what we are not aware of.

ADHD coaching has allowed me – even encouraged me – to feel safe in examining what my own intersectionality means to me, and in achieving enlightenment and change that could never have been possible without the overriding understanding of how my brain worked, and how I was experiencing the world around me.

My work and lived experience in the LGBT+ (lesbian, gay, bisexual, transgender, and other identities) community made me very aware, almost painfully, of the way I experienced privilege compared to others. Being gender non-conforming, assigned female at birth, and generally female-passing meant I could choose when to confront, and when to hide, my own intersectional identity.

Coaching allowed me the space to work out that, when I was loudly declaring 'You can use any pronouns for me, just try it out, it's okay if it doesn't work', I was really working super hard to manage other people's discomfort – and discounting mine.

Coaching allowed me the time to come back again and again to why I couldn't go to 'female founders' or 'women in business' events; to work through my strong, ADHD-attached feelings about social justice and fighting for 'others' in that space, and to conclude that actually, I *was* the 'other', and the notion I might be rejected or unwelcome was keeping me in a loop of seeking acceptance...which wouldn't be meaningful to me, even if it did come.

SUZY JACKSON, THE TECHNICOLOUR PROJECT,
ADHD SPECIALIST COACH

Suzy's account of examining their needs in specific situations demonstrates the important trust and safety that can be created when we are invited to think about our intersectionality and how this works for us in specific situations. Suzy also demonstrates how coaching acts as a pause to help them become aware of what is happening in a specific moment. Part of ADHD coaching is to extend this practice of pausing beyond the coaching space in order to connect to ourselves and our needs habitually.

3. LOVE AND CONNECTION TO OURSELVES

Step 1: Systematic pausing

I have an entire life of skipped-over emotions, achievements, events, relationships, experiences, TV awards, precious moments, always rushing to the next thing.

I can fall into the seductive trap of hyperfocusing on a result. Before I understood my ADHD, if I was writing, I hyperfocused. I didn't know how to restart a task, judge how well I was doing, and move on to something else. Like many of my ADHD clients, this was my strategy – push through, keep pushing, keep going, don't stop. I knew, in action, with people waiting, tight deadlines, I could achieve the impossible. If I slowed down, I was scared I would be a ship in the doldrums, without the wind. Listless, depressed, at the mercy of all that blue sea and sky. Waiting, waiting, waiting for a sign of something, a stirring of interest.

AVON HARPLEY, ADHD SPECIALIST COACH

Pausing is hard. We're all managing busy schedules, and sometimes it can feel impossible to just put the brakes on. And that's exactly why pausing is a radical act for those of us with what Dr Ned Hallowell (2019) calls 'Ferrari brains with bicycle brakes'. Learning to monitor the Ferrari and strengthen the bike brakes takes a lot of practice.

The very concept of 'pausing' may itself conjure up limiting 'I can't' beliefs. Here, Lizzie talks about her limiting beliefs:

If I get down to the beliefs about pausing, I think one was, 'If I pause, I won't be doing something and if I'm not doing something, I will be failing in some way.'

And the other belief was, 'When I pause, my mind doesn't sit still anyway so what's the point? And if I try, I sit there, frustrated and feeling bad because I just can't be still.'

LIZZIE BENTLEY BOWERS, EXECUTIVE COACH AND ADHD SPECIALIST COACH

In Lizzie's honesty about pausing, we can see a number of things at play: a need to keep going by doing because doing keeps us safe from failing. While this is a story, the fear of getting frustrated is very much because of the way we are wired and many of us will actively avoid frustration and the emotional dysregulation that shuts our brains down as a result.

The anticipation of frustration is often based on attempts to 'rest' or 'slow down' because we were told to and feel we should. This is 'importance' rather than connecting to why it might be important to us and therefore 'interesting'. As we have seen already, if we are not interested then we will struggle to do anything! Pausing for us may be associated with painful experiences of boredom or shame at failing to enjoy supposedly relaxing things like yoga or even holidays!

The key to pausing is to make it brief to begin with! Then it's about getting clear on the why, and that a pause can be adapted to suit our needs in any situation. First, we will need to connect with the personal felt benefits of pausing in order to get interested in applying it in different ways. Here, Lizzie talks about how coaching helped her to connect to her 'why':

> Coaching helped me to identify why pausing was important to me and understand what I would get if I paused. When it comes to pausing in coaching, I was like 'But I'm good at coaching, so it's fine.' Whereas now I'm like, 'Okay, well, what's important about this is that I'm even better at the things that I want to be good at if I do these pauses.' That's a powerful reframe. And I also want to be well, as far as I possibly can be. I want to be able to run, I want to be able to lift weights, I want to be able to keep up with my boys and my husband. And if I don't pause, I will burn out again and again and again. And that's what I understood from coaching and experimenting with pausing.
>
> LIZZIE BENTLEY BOWERS, EXECUTIVE COACH
> AND ADHD SPECIALIST COACH

We can see how Lizzie has changed her narrative from surviving to winning. Before the narrative was, 'Nothing bad happened so it's fine' but now it is, 'What more could I learn, if I pause?'

Your coach can facilitate pausing within the session and help you notice the benefits after the pause. Your coach can also help to bring your attention to situations in which you have paused, the benefits of the pause, and the strengths you used to pause.

Once you have worked with a coach who can help you figure out the best ways of pausing in different situations, you can establish experiments for pausing. This can be in the moment, after the moment, or scheduled into a routine or structure which can be trialled for a short period. All pausing is good – whether we are pausing to figure out moments of difficulty or moments of brilliance.

Here, Avon Harpley talks about the power that pausing has had on her life and recalls a powerful moment when she was invited to give an answer and instead paused and resisted:

I have learned that if I take the time to pause and tune in, my ADHD is a barometer to my environment, internal state, the quality of my thinking, the quality of my life, and how I am spending my time.

Recently, I was asked for a quick tip for working with ADHD clients, something that will help them solve their procrastination or stay focused. I paused, a life-changing act for me, and reflected. I used to believe that it would be that simple, if I could only find the perfect productivity tip to transform my life. I have learned instead to embrace feeling uncomfortable, frustrated, lost. I learned that some things can't be rushed. This is not a destination to reach but a way of life. Here you can find awareness, self-advocacy, peace, joy, compassion, acceptance, freedom, creativity, fun, connection, and support, and fall back in love with life again. These are the real riches.

From this place you can create a life that works for you and your quirky, contradictory, wonderful brain.

AVON HARPLEY, ADHD SPECIALIST COACH

In Avon's example, she was being invited to be the Rescuer drama position with a quick-fix answer to ADHD. By pausing, she realized that there isn't a quick fix and resisted the invitation to rescue the client. She tuned into what she knows, even withholding when the answer felt uncomfortable.

Pausing helps us to move away from rushing to, 'What is the *right* answer?' to, 'What is *my* right answer? What is true for me?'. Pausing helps bring us back to ourselves and our felt experience but in order to experience the kind of transformational learning Lizzie and Avon have had, we may need ways or steps during the pause to figure out what is going on for us.

Emotional granularity

(Barrett 2017) – Pinpointing and naming our feelings (even if there are many to pinpoint!).

Awareness of our physical state can help us identify feelings and meet our needs. Paying attention to our bodily sensations, and the feelings and needs they may be indicating, is part of how we can journey through recovery from not knowing ourselves to moving forward from an empowered place. When we can identify our needs and find ways to meet them, we are empowered to make choices and live our lives on our own terms!

However, one of the hardest differences to accept can be our emotionality, our dysregulation, and the intensity of our feelings. Some of us will openly express our emotions and some of us will have learned to hold them in and hide them, as we saw in Chapter 1. We may have found ways to daydream about new and imagined or nostalgic places rather than staying present. Many of us can feel dissociated from our bodies and what they are telling us. When we hide, ignore, or dissociate from our bodily sensations which indicate our feelings, over time we become disconnected from our bodies and what they are telling us (van der Kolk, 2014). Nathan describes his understanding of how the culture of masculinity affected his experience of ADHD and his relationship to his feelings, and how this went on to affect him as an adult:

Social norms and expectations for a white cis male growing up in the 80s and 90s in New Zealand didn't welcome high emotion and sensitivity. Each year of school the message got louder: boys don't behave like this! Many things could set me off, a new task in class, a new lesson, getting something wrong in class, engaging with other students. Bolts of anxiety and emotion would strike through my nervous system.

Significant spikes of overwhelm were a daily occurrence that year in school; some days it was impossible to hold it in and it was expressed in tears.

Reflecting now on that era of growing up, if I had expressed overwhelm as aggression, it would've ironically been considered far more appropriate and normal for a boy.

I thought there was something broken within me, so I began to close things off, finding ways to silo and avoid situations, paths, and relationships that would create an emotional overwhelm. That 11-year-old no longer had a voice. I lived life with an expectation of rejection if I showed my true self. Don't be vulnerable, and be sure to mask who I am.

As an adult, my life was lived at arm's length as a way to keep me from experiencing something I thought I might not be able to handle, or worse, exposing myself fully to someone who would ultimately reject me.

This survival mode revealed itself most in intimate relationships. I sought short-term relationships, yet longed for something far more intimate and long term. For me, emotional intimacy was fraught with danger and overwhelm, where I would no longer be able to mask.

I genuinely felt something was wrong with me, holding myself together daily, having to mask so much to get by. How could I sustain a long-term relationship? How could I be a good husband or father?

NATHAN

The clarity and vulnerability in Nathan's words is inspiring but we can see how difficult this would have been for his 11-year-old self to appreciate given the culture of masculinity of the time. Many of us will have grown up thinking that emotionality is a sign of weakness and will have taken decades trying to keep it down and out of sight. It can be scary to suddenly start acknowledging feelings that we've spent our whole lives trying to ignore.

We may also begin to realize that early experiences in normative and conforming environments like school were not designed to support or encourage our emotionality. Part of healing ourselves is about integrating ADHD into who we are in all our identities rather than hiding and compartmentalizing.

The problem with all survival techniques is that they work in the short term. By not paying attention to our body and our feelings, we can go even faster and get more stuff done (or so we think) so the idea of pausing or even talking about feelings will often lead to resistance in coaching. As ADHDers, our 'now, not now' sense of time and the intensity with which we feel things will make tolerating the discomfort very challenging to begin with.

Alternatively, we may try to think through and rationalize our feelings in order to find certainty without connecting to our felt experiences. When asked about feelings in coaching, we will often give a cognitive response or start taking the conversation in another direction. This is often unconscious to begin with but the coach can help to gently bring our bodies into our awareness.

The important thing with feelings is to approach them and our bodily sensations with curiosity and love rather than fear – this can take a while to reframe! The idea is that we become the 'coach' or 'nurturer' (see the Winning Triangle in Chapter 1) to our felt experience. We will need to have the bigger picture on why being able to identify feelings is an important skill as well as a really clear understanding of why it's harder for us. This changes the idea from a scary or shaming 'should' to 'interest'.

These are the five 'whys' of emotional granularity:

1. Slowing down to feel our bodily sensations and feelings can be an important process supporting self-acceptance. Accepting that our feelings are valid and worth listening to starts the move towards self-validation discussed in the next section.

2. Listening to our bodies and feelings helps us to make decisions (something we often struggle with) and to connect to what is important to us rather than what is interesting in the moment.

3. By knowing how we feel, we are able to eventually identify what we might need, changes we may want to make in order to support ourselves in thriving.

4. It is very difficult to thrive sustainably without being able to use Challenger in the Winning Triangle which protects our peace or our 'thrive'. The Challenger position often means being able to feel when something isn't okay for you so that you can assert your boundaries.

5. When we can get granular on how we feel, it can be a very important source of our power.

Here Nathan talks about the power of learning to sit with his emotions and what this has led to in his life:

Coaching helped me navigate, reflect, and open up to my emotions – something I had been pushing down since I was 11.

I learned to consciously employ them, situation by situation. Kindness was a big strength for me and played a pivotal part. For the first time in my life I began to use that strength on myself, and on my emotions day to day.

It created a shift not only in self-perception but in consciously changing how I engaged with the world. How to mask and fit in no longer came first; instead, I prioritized consciously looking for ways to meet my emotional needs, to help bring certainty to my day. This felt so alien, but with daily work scenarios that would normally mean high anxiety and loss of cognition, for example, speaking in public, they changed in my mind and had more space.

I was finally being open about who I was, how I was feeling, and what my needs were – not just at an intellectual level but at a gut level, a deep emotional level. Affirming daily that that 11-year-old boy was never broken. I was never broken.

Coaching shifted how I saw high sensitivity and emotion; it can be a superpower.

Embracing emotion helped my brain function better, with less anxiety and tiredness.

Even taking the risk of opening up fully in an intimate relationship, initially experiencing tightness in my chest and in my head, internal dialogues calling a stop to it all and all the other manifestations of years of layered self-programmed resistance, this work helped me finally let go of the mask and be completely vulnerable.

I wasn't rejected; instead there was a deeper connection.

The work has been worth it. That 11-year-old boy would be proud!

NATHAN

We can see how not understanding how we are different can lead to defaulting to others at the expense of hearing ourselves and our voices. The negative voice that we have internalized may mean we have little to no confidence in listening to ourselves. We may not trust our emotions, seeing them as momentary tsunamis not to be taken seriously. By starting to hear ourselves again, we start to validate our thoughts and feelings instead of continuing to ignore and repress them.

Learning to recover our trust in ourselves, self-validate, and resist the spiral into self-doubt or shame can require a number of processes which involve both strengths work and emotional granularity:

1. By learning how to be successful with our differences (experimenting with the ADHD lens in different situations) we start to be able to rely on ourselves, which builds our confidence.

2. By learning how to start spotting the strengths in what we do, we build a language with which to talk about ourselves

positively and an alternative lens with which to appreciate ourselves and that we are worth protecting.

3. In order to tap into 'being', we need to start engaging with our bodily sensations and labelling our emotions (emotional granularity) so that we can be clear about what we feel and what we need.

4. When we start to systematically listen to our feelings and needs and actively meet or get help to meet those unmet needs, we shift from powerless drama positions to winning more often. We may start to disrupt survival behaviours and meet our needs differently.

In this next excerpt, Lizzie Bentley Bowers talks about what has changed for her as a result of getting curious about her emotions:

Since having coaching I notice that when I'm 'in sensitivity' I narrate it differently. So I'll be saying things to myself like, 'Okay, we're in it now. Okay, I think that probably is a valid piece of "upsetness". We're going to be here for a while, so how about we distract ourselves with this thing or that thing?'

And I now choose mostly different distractions. So a glass of wine and food are much less on the distraction list than they used to be. I can talk myself around it in a different way. And I might still have the same kind of distraction solution or I might say, you know, how can I just have a conversation with myself that is much more along the lines of a coaching conversation? I may be curious about support or I might challenge myself, but what I do a lot less is try and make it go away and pretend it's not happening, or feel shame about it.

LIZZIE BENTLEY BOWERS, EXECUTIVE COACH
AND ADHD SPECIALIST COACH

We can see that Lizzie has begun to challenge old ways of managing emotional intensity. Until we have started validating our strengths, feelings, and needs, our ability to self-advocate can be tentative, unclear, rigid, or incomplete. The rush to self-advocate may be actively encouraged from our workplaces before we have had support and time to build clarity.

For some, the clarity of our feelings or the knowledge of how we are different is enough to find our voices and start communicating needs. For others, the practice of using our voice to express our feelings and needs may take mini experiments or rehearsals or scripts. Once we experience brave steps that don't lead to the perceived annihilation, we tend to grow bolder!

Once we are good at listening to and challenging ourselves to pause, we not only spot feelings but also the stories we are holding about ourselves. When we are clear on our differences, we start to loosen the negativity. If we want to truly move forward, we can't just spot bad stories; we need to replace them with honesty about our challenges and clarity about our strengths – strengths that were often buried.

4. SELF-VALIDATION WHEN WE ARE HIGHLY SITUATIONAL

Neurodivergent brains have spiky cognitive profiles. This means that the difference between our strengths and our challenges is more pronounced regardless of where a profile might sit in relation to average. For example, my verbal processing is around 125 (where the average is 95–105) but my short-term memory is 89. The difference between 125 and 89 is significant. Again, if we haven't understood this difference, we tend to focus on our challenges and not our strengths. This means that we have often found accepting ourselves very difficult as our attention is trained on to focus on our difficulties.

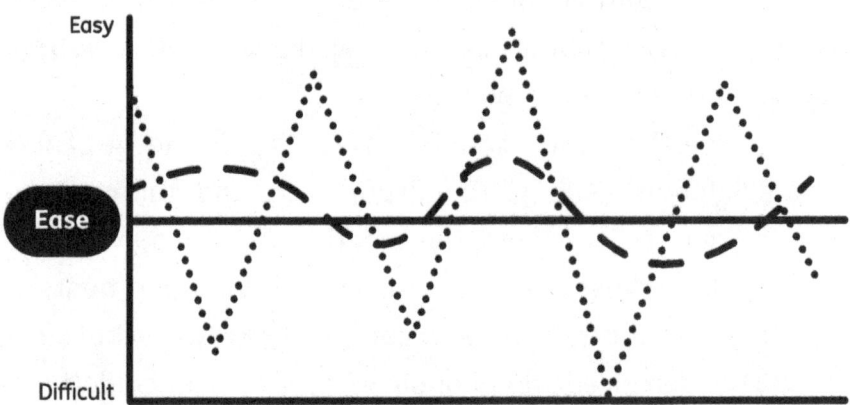

Figure 2.5: Spiky profiles

Source: Adapted from Dr Nancy Doyle's Spiky Profile model (2019). © 2024 by Gold Mind Academy.

This is made harder if we are diagnosed later in life and may have some deeply ingrained narratives on how we think about ourselves based on frustrating and disappointing experiences (such as those highlighted in the previous section), where we couldn't fully understand what was going on for us.

Strengths that we do experience are often dismissed, discounted, or greatly overshadowed by our perceived challenges. Not only may we have minimal language with which to talk about our personal strengths, we can also be incredibly resistant to talking about ourselves positively.

We may never have been encouraged to talk positively about ourselves. Our parents, who are also likely to be neurodivergent, may not have modelled talking positively about themselves or about us. For many of us, depending on our marginalization, making ourselves smaller may have been encouraged. For others with more privilege, self-deprecation and positioning themselves as 'ordinary' may have also been encouraged in order to uphold systems of privilege (Khan, 2009; Reeves & Friedman, 2024).

Finally, if our ADHD lens has only been narrated through a clinical lens, as a disorder or a disease, we are even less likely to see any aspect of it as positive. In fact, we may have lost all sense of what's good about us.

We have so far talked about strengths as 'anything we feel we are good at'. If we were to identify any, they may be aligned to our cognitive strengths. For example, before understanding neurodivergence I would have been able to describe myself as good at talking especially when learning languages but my attention would have then been drawn to diminish this because of what was a fear of public speaking which was largely based on problems with remembering speeches.

The VIA (Values in Action) Character Strengths are a helpful reframe of strengths. Rather than seeing strengths as something you have or don't have, character strengths are all within us and available for us to express in any given situation. They can serve as a way of framing success that goes beyond chasing the dopamine of achievement, which often feels empty the moment we have achieved it. VIA strengths can be a way of connecting to our importance and therefore our positive interest.

Our strengths can spark our interest-based nervous systems to start seeing ourselves through a new lens: 'Who am I being when...', not the default dopamine-seeking, 'How many things have I ticked off?' A good place to begin is by taking 'noticings' and linking them to our strengths:

Example:

Coachee: I noticed that my attention was starting to slide by 12.30 today so rather than ploughing on and getting slower and more frustrated, I walked home for lunch and did ten minutes of yoga.

Coach: What strengths do you notice?

Coachee: I guess I used self-regulation to notice my attention and pivot... What does prudent mean again?

Coach: Making careful decisions and planning with your future in mind.

Coachee: Yeah, I guess I was prudent then. I have never thought of it like that as I would often see leaving work as failure. I guess I was being kind to myself too because walking and

yoga really helped me and I remembered to eat which sometimes doesn't happen till I'm dysregulated.

By having a new framework for success around who we are, there
is a lot more to appreciate and it can invite new ways of thinking.
It can be really hard for us to plan ahead and think about our
future self, but not impossible when we have a new framework
for success.

In the example above, that ADHDer is using strengths which
are newer to them, but once they have a language of appreciation they can start to see things differently. Instead of slogging
away at a marathon and getting frustrated and coming home
hangry, they took a pause, met some needs, and came back
energized.

Strengths work can be very energizing! Here Elisabeth talks
about how understanding neurodivergence led her to realize she
was 'okay'. As a result of strengths work in community, she can
identify how she experiences strengths and attributes them to
her neurodivergence:

I only realized I was autistic when I completed an online
profiling tool at the age of 60. And I only realized that I had
ADHD traits when I took the Gold Mind Academy course
on ADHD a couple of years later. Discovering both of these
things in my sixties has been quite an experience: what has
sat uncomfortably with me over many years as 'being different' from other women I now understand as being okay.

Although it feels like the nature of my strengths and

challenges shifts around a little, here is what they seem to me now:

- Creativity: I am creative – I pull ideas from multiple places to create something new. This comes through in my writing, coaching work, and the eco group I've created and led in my village.

- Self-development, learning, and knowledge: I love to learn about myself, everything to do with my coaching, what we can do to support the environment. And I enjoy sharing that knowledge with others. It's probably what influenced the choice of my first career in information and knowledge management. I knew both of these things before I found out about my neurodivergence. But I now appreciate how my creativity is an ADHD strength, and that the curiosity that drives my learning is spiky.

- Leadership and teamwork: It was only in one of the recent peer-coaching sessions with Gold Mind Academy, exploring peak experiences, that I realized how big a part my leadership and teamwork skills are playing in my environmental work too. I'm always surprised by how reluctant so many people are to take the lead in making things happen, and how easy it is for me to do so.

- Tenacity and organizational skills: Last but not least is my tenacity and my ability to organize and get things done, which come from the autistic side of my being. I used to get frustrated by how slow other people could be to respond to my initiatives, or about how I would need to adapt my well-laid plans. My work and life experiences have taught me to be more relaxed about this; to recognize that change is inevitable and can be for the better; to let plans evolve over time. I use my creative strength and enjoy looking out for and using 'open door' opportunities.

This increased understanding of my own autism and ADHD has had a dramatic impact on my coaching.

As coaches, we 'sit' with empathy, with our clients' emotions first. I feel that my empathy has grown with my understanding as a parent, and with my self-compassion as an individual who is neurodivergent.

It feels as if I've missed many opportunities to understand my strengths and challenges in life. I'm sad that I was not able to explore these further with my parents before they died. But I am revelling in the opportunity to celebrate and lean into my strengths more and to be self-compassionate about, advocate for, and support my challenges better.

ELISABETH GOODMAN (PCC – ICF), RIVERRHEE
CONSULTING, COACH, AUTHOR, AND ACTIVIST

Elisabeth talks about the frustration she had with others who couldn't do what she could do and how she now understands this as a strength in her rather than a deficit in others. Interestingly, Elisabeth notes that her capacity to be empathetic with others has grown as a direct result of being empathetic to herself and her understanding of her needs. This is a huge gift in strengths work; when we start to see our strengths, we can show up differently for others.

A good ADHD coach will invite you to see the strengths in your stories and your actions as well as during the coaching session. It is important that the coach is not continuously validating you, as this reinforces the constant seeking for external validation. Instead, they should be continuously inviting you to notice your strengths. We need to learn how to see our strengths for ourselves and truly experience them, in order to get the clarity Elisabeth demonstrates. Whenever we use strengths in coaching, we produce a visual or we encourage you, the client, to find a visual of the VIA strengths on your phone. Engaging in strengths work without a prompt will end up with a very surface level response where you may feel tested or ashamed about what you can't remember!

Elisabeth mentions that her strengths feel as if they 'shift around a little'. This is because our strengths and challenges are highly situational; they will depend on the task we are trying to do, the environment we are in (including the people we are with), and how well supported a version of us shows up to the situation.

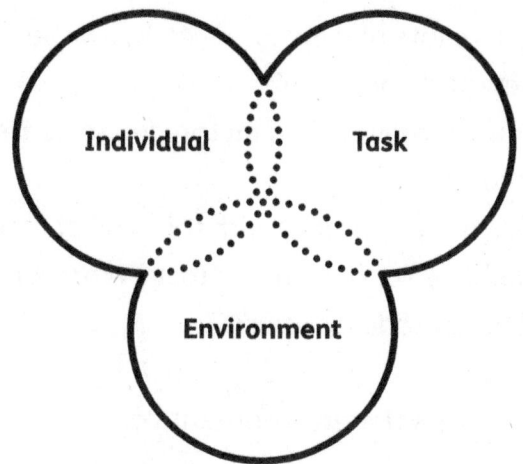

Figure 2.6: Situational variability

Source: Amanda Kirby's TIE model (2021), Do-IT Profiler.

Individual – to what extent were you supported to do the task?

- How well were your physical needs met? Sleep, nutrition, exercise, medicines?
- How well were your emotional needs met? Mood, space to process and regulate?
- Where were your dopamine levels? What had you already achieved that day?
- Was there anything breaking your attention? Worries, distractions, overwhelm?
- What is the story you are telling yourself about the task and about you? Strengths?

Task – what kind of task?

- Were you interested in the task negatively or positively?
- What else made it easier or harder to do?

- Were there lots of steps? Did you know the steps or were they new and uncertain?
- How much time had you factored in to do this task? Was this accurate?!
- What is your experience with this kind of task?
- Did you have support in this task? What kind of support would have made it easier?

Environment – was the environment conducive to you in the task?

- Who were you with and what effect were they having on you? Did you feel safe? Did you feel energized? Was there clear communication?
- What was the impact of the physical environment on your senses and your ability to get the task done? Light, noise, temperature, smell, and so on?

Here is an example of how we might use the situational variability model in coaching. Note that again, we would recommend drawing the model with a visual prompt to hang your insights on.
Example:

Coachee: Well, yesterday I managed to write about 2500 words before 3pm and then I had a complete disaster trying to get into my Government Gateway to sort some tax stuff out.

Coach: The tax task sounds very frustrating but I am also hearing a huge achievement in writing this many words by 3pm. What helped you to write so many words?

Coachee: Oh I don't know, I guess I just hit an easy section.

Coach: So the section you were writing was easy...what else? Perhaps if we look at the situational variability circles you may get some more ideas...

Coachee: Well, I think the key is that I managed to start at 9.30am. I wrote the day out with timings for my breaks and lunch, which felt like wasting time at 9am but I think it helped me to get going, seeing the end. Then I wrote little tasks I was allowed to do in my breaks and also how many words I had to do in each burst... I am not medicated at the moment as I have a bit of a bug, but I definitely got seven or eight hours' sleep the night before. I think it helped because I was hitting these mini targets which then helped me to keep going on the third stint. I mean, I was definitely starting to scroll on my phone and get sidetracked but it was okay as I had hit my target. Yeah, I think my targets are getting more realistic. I was also listening to fast-paced music with no words, which really helped me to pace my actions. When I felt myself getting restless and distracted, I went to have lunch and I realized I had got really cold just sitting around so I had a shower and this always helps as my mind just wanders in the shower and I always feel really restored.

Coach: Wow! So there was so much nuance on how you are being successful and you started with 'I just hit an easy section'. What strengths are you now seeing in this detail?

Coachee: Errm, I guess I was getting perspective when I wrote the tasks out and set targets, and maybe it was love for myself because I noticed I was cold and I took time to have a shower.

Coach: You said that your targets are getting more realistic. What do you notice there?

Coachee: I guess, judgement? And love of learning because I'm trying to learn from when they have not been realistic.

Coach: What are you learning about yourself in this?

Coachee: I am starting to know how I work and that a lot of it is trial and error but it is getting better.

Coach: Great! I wonder what made the tax task so hard then, looking at the model?

Coachee: Yeah, well I am realizing that I thought I would engage with it for 30 minutes but in reality the whole thing took nearly two hours, which is clearly why I was getting so frustrated. I am glad I put it at the end of the day though, because at least I had written my words.

Coach: So you managed to stick at it for nearly two hours?

Coachee: Yeah! And I did eventually find my username and recreate a password, even if I still haven't managed to authorize my accountant to sort out my tax yet.

Coach: And what strengths were you using to stick at it and get as far as you did?

Coachee: I guess I was self-regulating enough. Actually, my dog needed to go out and was making it pretty clear so there was an involuntary break, which probably helped me to keep going. But I think I was understanding why it was hard for me, whereas before I would be in this place of shame and judgement, like, 'Why can't you do what everyone else can?' I think this actually helped me and I knew that all the steps were frustrating. All the waiting for automated options and still not getting to speak to a human on the Government Gateway site. Even when I clicked the additional needs link I got so many options and was so overwhelmed but I just thought this is a 'them' thing not a me thing. They need to understand why things are harder like I do...so yeah, if I think about it, even the tax disaster was an improvement on years gone by where I would have ended up crying on the floor. I am further along and can pick it up on Monday.

Coach: And what difference does knowing that make?

Coachee: It makes me feel hopeful that things can get better and that I am not stuck or wrong. It makes me think that hard things like writing a book and sorting my tax out can be achieved, and that makes me feel free.

By looking through a lens of situational variability we can appreciate and understand the nuance of situations which start off as very black and white: 'I wrote 2500 words (good) and had a complete disaster with the Government Gateway tax issue (bad).'

The nuance that the model invites can stop us from attributing success to luck: 'I guess I just hit an easy section.' This is a shortcut from our default brain. These shortcuts often lead to limiting beliefs and narratives about ourselves. If these aren't challenged, they play a huge part in how we tackle new tasks. If we don't get under the surface of ADHD, our brain starts taking shortcuts and making 'I can't...' statements, which hold us back. Not only do we remain stuck, but we perpetuate an image of disability as 'fixed' rather than situational. Equally, if we don't pay attention to our strengths and understand what environments and tasks support them, we can't rely on and trust them.

I have learned to do more of the things that come easily to me, and that there are some tasks I will never do by myself, but can complete in a day, with a friend.

Most importantly, I see my strengths as something to be used, not left hidden and forgotten. This is ongoing learning. I, like many others, have always focused on what I couldn't do, on weaknesses to be improved.

AVON HARPLEY, ADHD SPECIALIST COACH

Appreciating the nuance of the 'situational' nature of our ADHD can take time and a number of chances to think through different moments of difficulty and triumph. We tend to be able to analyse our moments of difficulty because they are interesting, whereas analysing our wins is important and we may need more help to connect to why it is important to us (and therefore interesting!).

Often when asked about wins at the beginning of a coaching session, we will quickly list a number of achievements and then get straight to the pain point – because it's more interesting! However, it is worth delving into the successes *and* the pain points because there is often a lot of situational nuance to be found in positive examples which we can learn from if we slow down to reflect.

5. SELF-ADVOCACY

When we get interested and clear about how situations can bring out strengths or challenges we see choice.

> Should we just sit here hoping that one day the world will recognize the needs for the neurodiverse? Or, could we choose to acknowledge the self through a self-compassionate lens and change our surroundings instead of our brains?
>
> **GARETH DAKIN**

Once the self-criticism is loosened through strength (considering the normative systems and the ADHD lens), then self-compassion and forgiveness can grow. We start to see people and environments more clearly and we eventually realize there is choice, as Gareth mentions above. Once we have clarity and certainty to be nurturing to our vulnerabilities we realize we have to protect ourselves and this involves being assertive.

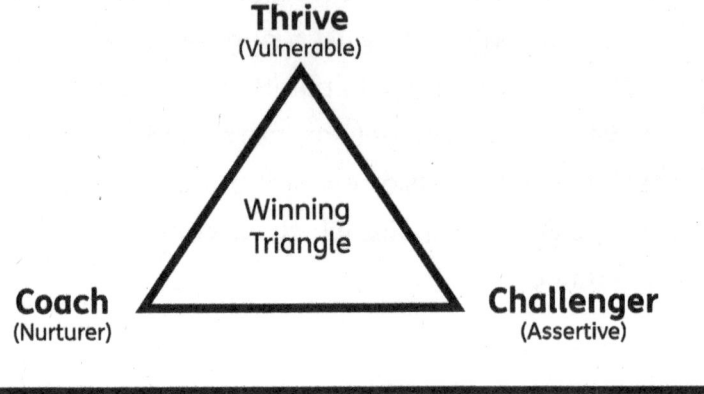

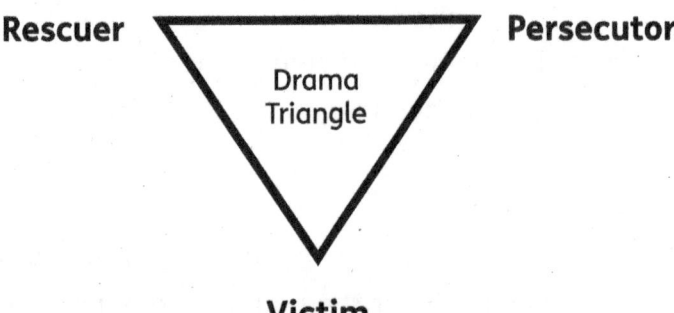

Figure 2.7: The Drama and Winning Triangles

Source: Adapted from Stephen Karpman's Drama Triangle (1968) and David Emerald's Empowerment Dynamic (2005). © 2024 by Gold Mind Academy.

Here, a coaching client describes how coaching supported her in becoming assertive with a work situation that was not serving her well:

I am now able to catch when I am falling into a 'right and wrong' story. My own right and wrong story is normally some version of where there is a good way and there is a bad way – a bad way that is my fault. I wrestled with this false dichotomy in work and it inevitably escalated into a situation where my mental health was poor and I felt stuck in the cycle. I was so afraid of what would happen if I truly shared how much I was struggling.

Confronted by the vicious cycle, I was able to spot some of the stories I was telling myself and take steps that felt scary and radical – but ultimately affirming. I called in sick and was honest that it was mental health. In my back-to-work conversation I did not blame myself or the underlying clinical condition, but I clearly stated that work was exacerbating it and shared with my line manager their part in the cycle. And I did those things in a way that was authentic to me; it was direct but it was also kind.

My coach had been supporting me to pause and assess my feelings and needs for months and this was probably the most significant pause I've ever taken. There was a lightbulb moment before I made the sick call where I literally went through what I had practised – noticing how I was feeling, thinking about what was causing it – and in that pause I finally caught the unmet needs that needed addressing. (Another great sign of coaching is that I can hear my coach calling me out on the 'finally' and asking me to offer myself some compassion for all the reasons that it might take a long time to get to this point.)

There is much to celebrate from that back-to-work conversation and it was in coaching that I really landed that success and realized how many coaching tools I had reached for without even noticing – not just in the conversation itself but in the planning of it, the timing of it, and all the little ways I was able to optimize the conditions of the call and maximize my strengths.

The full power of my strengths was vital as it honestly felt like one of the first times I authentically shared that I needed something. Years of masking have taught me that I'll be praised for being easy going, and that sweet praise is far easier to get at than my actual preferences. It was in coaching that I rehearsed finding my preferences and I no longer believe that it is a core personality trait of mine that 'I just don't mind, I like going with the flow.'

ANONYMOUS

In this last paragraph, the coaching client is clear that her strengths helped her shift from external validation to self-validation, which then gave her the choice to challenge the person who she once relied on to validate her. She also talks about how she had begun to use coaching tools without even noticing. This is where the new ways of being become easeful and automated and we start to be ourselves with less effort and fear!

6. PUTTING IT ALL TOGETHER – YOU ON PURPOSE

Perhaps the best way to illustrate the power of ADHD coaching is to give an example of a change of narrative:

I was recently in central London on my way to deliver Neurodiversity Deep Dive Training to a corporate company. I had been told the building was 'to the left' of a central train station. I had pictured it in my head and felt clear about where I was going and I had booked a hotel nearby. When I got to the station and found the building to the left, I realized that 'to the left' depends on whether you are facing the station or not. The building I had envisaged was not it and I felt the panic and frustration rise as I realized how many possible buildings I may have to try and how little time I had left to figure this out.

Rather than let the panic give way to tears and persecution of myself for my lack of planning and attention to detail, I began narrating in my head and giving non-judgemental explanation of how I was in this situation: *You have not researched the exact location of the venue because your 'now/ not now' time perception meant it wasn't interesting enough at the time. Last night you worked late and thought you knew where the building was anyway. This is a situation you don't practise regularly and you have been caught out. Now your brain is flooding with frustration and fear that you won't get there on time. If you don't breathe and stay calm, your brain will shut down, so keep breathing and let's walk around the other side of the station...*

Not only did I find the right building but thanks to my creativity and zest, I also managed to weave this very live example into the training I delivered that day. I was able to describe what would have happened before I had done a lot of coaching work around my ADHD – I may well have been in tears and made panicked phone calls and come into the training dishevelled, late, and apologetic. Instead, I was calm and was also able to improvise when there were problems with the tech set up. Rather than be ashamed that I couldn't figure out the tech and was somehow inadequate, I was clear that I was being hired for my training and neurodiversity expertise and that the company would have an expert or someone with more tech expertise than me.

KATIE FRIEDMAN

This feels like 'You on purpose': clarity on my strengths and challenges, ability to manage challenges in the moment and use the struggles to help others, ability to delegate, ask for help, and take responsibility for and set boundaries around my remit. If I imagine 'You on purpose' in the context of the Ditzler model, I am now operating in the central zone: who I really am (in all my strengths and challenges). There is honesty where before there was masking and pretending; there is neutral narration, which keeps my brain online rather than the self-persecution that shuts it down in moments of difficulty. By knowing that I am an awesome trainer and course creator who uses strengths like humour, honesty, love, and bravery, I am accepting of the things that I find more difficult (like planning logistics and managing a new computer and synching it to a company system when the company system is playing up).

'You on purpose' means that we are able to stay regulated or come back there much faster. This is not only hugely beneficial for our mental health, but also for our physical health. Doing 'You on purpose' is empowering, and when we are empowered, we can have a positive influence on those around us. From this empowered place, we can make sustainable contributions that nourish both ourselves and those around us instead of draining us.

Honestly, I can't stop with the models – I bring them to my line management of others, to group meetings, to my part-ner! You don't need to say, 'Excuse me my love, we're in the Drama Triangle' but you can definitely use the shape of the model to point out what appears to be happening. This is far more empowering than when I previously was inclined to carry the whole responsibility for making things go well. That in itself is a multiplying gift of coaching – drama begets drama but thriving also begets thriving and I am modelling good behaviour!

I wouldn't want people to think that there is some kind of enlightenment moment and that everything is forever easy. I miss plenty of feelings and that's just being human, but the dial is shifting from ignoring my needs to a healthier balance of noticing and nurturing.

LILY EASTWOOD, ASSISTANT DIRECTOR

In the next chapter, we'll take a look at how you can get started with ADHD coaching and the things you will need to consider.

SUMMARY

Key takeaways
Understanding coaching:

- Definition and differentiation:
  - Coaching focuses on present and future growth, distinct from therapy, which often addresses past or present mental health issues.
  - Unlike mentoring, which involves guidance from a more experienced individual, coaching is a partnership between equals.
  - Coaching emphasizes self-directed growth, where clients set their own goals and work towards achieving them with the coach's support.

- ADHD coaching:
  - ADHD coaching is about deep-seated personal

development, understanding, and leveraging strengths, not just managing symptoms.

○ It involves helping clients define what thriving with ADHD looks like for them and supporting them in achieving this.

○ The coaching process includes competencies from both the International Coaching Federation and the Professional Association for ADHD Coaches.

ADHD Needs Pyramid:

- Building a foundation:
  ○ The ADHD Needs Pyramid illustrates the journey from survival to thriving, emphasizing building certainty, safety, and self-understanding.
  ○ ADHD coaching helps clients build a solid foundation of self-awareness and resilience, moving from survival mode to a state of thriving.
  ○ The Pyramid model aids in visualizing the steps needed to achieve personal growth and stability.

- Systematic pausing:
  ○ Learning to systematically pause can help manage the fast-paced ADHD brain and improve decision-making.
  ○ Pausing allows for reflection, which can lead to better emotional regulation and self-awareness.
  ○ Incorporating pauses into daily routines can help prevent burnout and increase overall well-being.

- Emotional granularity:
  - Understanding and naming emotions can enhance self-awareness and emotional regulation.
  - Emotional granularity helps in identifying needs and making informed decisions.
  - Developing this skill can lead to better self-advocacy and stronger personal boundaries.

- Recognizing normative systems:
  - Acknowledging and understanding how normative systems impact ADHD can help externalize rather than internalize challenges.
  - This awareness can foster self-acceptance and better navigation of societal expectations and biases.
  - It empowers individuals to advocate for themselves and create supportive environments.

- You on purpose:
  - Living 'You on purpose' means integrating ADHD into one's identity and leveraging strengths to thrive.
  - It involves moving from a place of survival to one of empowerment, where challenges are managed and strengths are highlighted.
  - This approach fosters a positive self-image and sustainable personal and professional growth.

REFLECTIVE QUESTIONS

1. How do you feel about focusing on your strengths instead of your 'deficits'? What might you need to consider to engage with this different approach?
2. What aspects of your life would you like to see improved through ADHD coaching?
3. In what ways could understanding your unique neurological makeup help you in all aspects of life?
4. How might developing a solid foundation of self-awareness impact your daily life?
5. What strategies could you use to incorporate systematic pausing into your routine, and what benefits might you notice?
6. How could learning to understand and name your emotions improve your self-awareness and decision-making?
7. In what ways might recognizing normative systems help you better advocate for yourself?
8. What does living 'You on purpose' mean to you, and how might it change your approach to daily life?
9. How do you currently view your strengths and challenges, and how might this perspective change through coaching?
10. What are some specific intentions you might like to set for yourself through ADHD coaching?

CHAPTER 3

Getting Started with an ADHD Coach

This chapter talks about the practical details around getting started with ADHD coaching and how to get the most out of the process. We will cover the following aspects:

1. Choosing a coach.
2. Funding, fees, and frequency.
3. Getting the most out of your coaching experience.
4. What if coaching isn't right for you right now?
5. Life beyond coaching.

CHOOSING A COACH

So how do you choose an ADHD coach?

Searching for a suitable coach can feel overwhelming. There is a huge amount of choice, and coaches will have different qualifications and approaches. In this chapter, we will outline what to look for and provide some helpful prompts when choosing your coach.

Work with a qualified coach

Terms such as clinical psychologists, or psychiatrists are protected categories but the term 'coach' is not. This means that the coaching industry is not regulated in the same way as the medical world. This has both positive and negative connotations. The positive is that people from all kinds of career trajectories can become a coach and bring their knowledge of the industry with them. However, it also means that there are many self-proclaimed 'ADHD coaches' who have little or no training. The ADHD coaching industry is booming and it's important to be aware of this when choosing a coach.

Given the lack of regulation in the coaching industry, it is strongly advised that you approach coaches who have completed certified ADHD-specific coach training accredited by one of the major coaching membership bodies (listed below). Being an ADHDer or holding a general coaching or life coaching qualification is not enough. While lived experience and general coach training can be valuable, they do not ensure a coach has the knowledge or tools to work effectively within a neurodivergent framework. ADHD-specific training is crucial for helping coaches integrate their understanding of ADHD both personally and professionally, and to apply it ethically and competently within a coaching framework. In the UK, a commonly recognised benchmark for coaching competence is a Level 5 qualification in Coaching or above. Alternatively, coaches may hold a formal credential awarded by an established coaching membership body, which serves as an equivalent qualification. Credentialing means the coach has demonstrated that they meet a set of agreed professional and academic standards. These typically include:

- Completion of a minimum number of accredited coach training hours (e.g. 60+ hrs for entry-level, 125+ hrs for intermediate, 200+ hrs for master)
- Documented coaching experience with real clients (e.g. 100+ hours for entry-level, 500+ for professional level, 2,500+ hrs for master)
- Participation in mentor coaching with a qualified mentor coach
- Ongoing supervision, Continued Professional Development or reflective practice
- Adherence to a code of ethics and core coaching competencies
- Successful completion of a credentialing exam to assess application of coaching knowledge and skills
- Look for coaches with one or more of the following credentials:

International Coaching Federation (ICF)

- Associate Certified Coach (ACC)
- Professional Certified Coach (PCC)
- Master Certified Coach (MCC)

European Mentoring and Coaching Council (EMCC)

- Practitioner
- Senior Practitioner

- Master Practitioner

Professional Association for ADHD Coaches (PAAC)

- Certified ADHD Coach Practitioner (CACP)
- Professional Certified ADHD Coach (PCAC)
- Master Certified ADHD Coach (MCAC)

Association for Coaching (AoC)

- Coach
- Professional Coach
- Master Coach

Even if your coach doesn't hold a credential yet, they should be able to give evidence of their training being accredited by one of the membership bodies AND be working towards one of the credentials listed above.

Within the ADHD coaching industry, there is a growing membership organization called the Professional Association for ADHD Coaches (PAAC). Why are these membership bodies important for you to know about? With the growth of the ADHD coaching profession, training institutions are also in higher demand, and there are several who do not meet any of the accreditation criteria of the above membership bodies.

Researching the coach

First, you will need to make contact with coaches you would like to meet for a 'discovery call'. This is a chance to meet your coach and for you to decide if you want to work with them. When researching coaches to meet, there are some questions you will want to have answered, ideally by simply browsing their website. If these answers are not readily available, it would be worth asking them via email before you meet:

- What can I expect in the coaching sessions? What is the structure?
- What can I expect in the coaching process with you over 12 sessions?
- How have you benefitted from ADHD coaching? What changes have you experienced personally?
- What have your clients said the value of ADHD coaching is?
- What specialist ADHD coach training have you completed and which coaching bodies accredited the training?
- What ongoing support (ADHD coach, coach supervisor, mentor coach, etc.) do you have for serving your clients?

The answers to these questions above will be a real indication of whether you are talking to a specialist or a generalist, and may indicate the quality of their training, their self-development, and the extent of their experience.

It's also completely appropriate to ask coaches for details about their data protection practices, insurance, supervision arrangements, and safeguarding protocols. In the UK, for example, professional coaches who collect client data should be registered with the Information Commissioner's Office (ICO). Depending on where you live, there may be a different body that oversees this, so it's worth checking what the equivalent is in your country.

You might have already asked about supervision as part of their ongoing development. But it's also important to know whether they have appropriate supervision protocols in place for ethical accountability and safeguarding, especially when things go wrong. Don't be afraid to ask about these things. A coach who is operating professionally should be able to easily confirm how they are meeting these responsibilities. It's another helpful sign that they take your safety, privacy, and the integrity of the coaching relationship seriously.

Even if a coach identifies as an ADHDer themselves, you still need to know what specialist ADHD coach training they have had. This training should be accredited by one or more of the professional coaching bodies, as mentioned earlier in this chapter. Beyond ADHD, a competent coach should also have a solid understanding of the broader neurodivergent landscape. ADHD frequently co-occurs with other neurotypes such as autism, dyslexia, and dyspraxia. This happens in more than half of diagnosed cases. A coach who recognises this overlap and is equipped to support a range of neurodivergent experiences will be better placed to understand the full picture of your lived reality. Accredited training alone is not the whole picture. You also want to know what ongoing support the coach receives to develop their own practice. This might include being part of a supervision group, working with a mentor coach, or engaging in a professional learning community. Asking about this is important. It tells you whether the coach is committed to continual development and is part of a wider professional network. Coaches who work in isolation without support may not be able to sustain their practice or offer you the same depth of insight. The most impactful coaches are usually those who stay connected, reflective, and well-resourced, both for themselves and for you.

The discovery call

As neurodivergent thinkers, we are more affected by and sensitive to the quality of relationships than other thinkers (Høglend, 2014; Wiseman & Tishby, 2017), which is why the relationship between you and your coach will be a crucial component as to whether the coaching is effective. It is therefore a good idea to take a few weeks to meet with different coaches before deciding who to go with. If the coaching is funded by Access to Work (available to UK residents) or your employer, you may be encouraged to go with an allocated coach, be pushed to use a certain provider, or feel as if you have less time to decide. Push back on this! It is really important that you have autonomy and take your time to consider who *you* want to work with.

One of the best predictors of coaching success is the quality of the relationship, or 'alliance,' between you and your coach. Coaching is a relational process, and that relationship needs to feel safe enough, collaborative, and spacious for you to do your best thinking. If, after a few sessions, it feels like the connection isn't quite right, it's okay to explore whether the relationship is still the best fit, even if you had originally planned to work together for a longer period. You are allowed to pause or end the coaching before the agreed timeline if it doesn't feel like it's working for you. If you're working with an employer or coaching provider, you should feel empowered to request a new coach. Many companies offer the option to change coach at least once without any additional cost. If your coaching is funded by your employer, remember: confidentiality still belongs to you. A good coach will be clear about this and help you navigate any competing agendas between you and your manager. Sometimes it can be helpful to involve your manager in an early conversation, facilitated by your coach in order to align expectations and support a shared understanding of the coaching focus.

ADHD coaches should request emergency contact details and possibly the contact details of therapists, GPs, and other clinicians in order to ensure that support is joined up if in an emergency. Coaches should explain in the discovery call that coaching is confidential; however, confidentiality may be broken if the coach believes that their client is an immediate danger to themselves or others. They should also mention that emergency services will be called at this point. The coach should state that coaching is a partnership with a client, but in the case of an emergency the coach may have to break this partnership and make decisions for the client in protecting life.

It is important to state that where there is significant ill-health or mental health conditions, these must be assessed and managed by an appropriate licensed clinician. While coaching can support us in understanding ourselves, it is not a substitute for medical or psychiatric treatment. Coaches are not qualified to diagnose or treat mental health conditions. If you are experiencing severe mental health symptoms or co-occurring conditions, it is critical to seek care from a licensed healthcare provider.

A good coach will ask you what you are hoping to get out of coaching overall and what matters to you. They will also be able to tell you what their approach is to ADHD coaching. It is quite normal to feel unclear about what you are hoping to get from coaching but you may be able to articulate what you would like to be different.

Some coaches will include important ethical questions in their discovery call (such as confidentiality, what coaching is, and how it differs from therapy or mentoring); others will include more of this in their intake forms or in the first coaching session. We call this 'contracting' or agreeing with your coach how you will work and what the boundaries of coaching are. The purpose of 'contracting' is to set up clarity and to ensure that trust and safety are being built from the outset. We will see in the section below on 'Getting the most out of your coaching experience' that contracting needs to be ongoing.

It is important to state that safety is relative and will depend on your specific intersectionality and your lived experience. It is therefore even more important that all elements of your experience are welcome in the coaching space, even if this is not something you have considered or particularly want to work on.

A good coach will ask you about your intersecting identities and how you would like to work with them in relation to your ADHD. Discussing your intersecting identity with your ADHD coach and exploring how you'll work with aspects of your identity that your coach does and doesn't identify with is often a good way of testing out if you feel you will be safe enough to work with this person. Consider how it will feel if you sense the coach's discomfort when you raise a topic which is directly related to your intersectional differences. If you don't get asked by the coach, we suggest you ask the coach, 'How do you work with differences in coaching?'

If you feel that you can only talk about ADHD and have to leave your racialization or your sexuality out because you sense the coach's fragility, you may find that you are having to work harder or not getting to your truth effectively. You need to know that your coach really understands ADHD while also being able to hold space for your specific lived experience, intersectionality, and any co-occurrences (diagnosed or not).

It's so interesting to me that I don't feel the need to ensure that my ADHD coach is queer like me... It's far more important that they're really, truly switched on to neurodivergence in all the ways it can show up. Because if you get that, everything else is...really clever listening!

SUZI JACKSON, TECHNICOLOUR, ADHD SPECIALIST COACH

The preference to have a coach who shares more areas of your intersectionality will depend on each individual and their experience and where they are in relation to their understanding of themselves. It is not always easy to find coaches with specific intersectional differences.

To find someone who is equipped in terms of racialized conversations, has an understanding of mental health and well-being, but also understands the neurodiverse brain, that's like a unicorn.

AISHA THOMAS, DIRECTOR OF REPRESENTATION
MATTERS, ADHD-INFORMED COACH

Aisha has actually become the unicorn she was looking for as she has trained as an ADHD coach who is also an anti-racism consultant and educator. We are lucky that Aisha is working with Gold Mind to help us ensure that our training equips coaches to work with difference effectively and that normativity is disrupted in our training in order to improve diversity and honour an intersectional lens.

After the discovery call

A coach should not put you on the spot to make decisions. Even if you feel the person is a great coach for you, we encourage you to delay the decision, *pause*, and give yourself some processing time. After the call ask yourself the following questions:

- How did I feel when I met them?
- Did I feel listened to and seen?
- Did I feel safe enough?
- Did I feel I was in the driving seat of the conversation?

FUNDING, FEES, AND FREQUENCY

One of the key pieces of information you will need to know is the cost of coaching. Coaches may advertise their coaching fees on their websites but most will have varying rates depending on whether you are self-funding, receiving state funding (such as the Access to Work scheme in the UK), or you are funded through your work.

Coaches may ask you who is funding the coaching. If you are, it is reasonable for you to be asked what you earn before they give you a coaching rate. If your work is funding the coaching, the coach may want to know more about your organization in order to provide a suitably equitable price for their service. For example, if you are working for the public sector, the price may be very different from what corporate companies are charged for executive coaching. There are often extra insurance costs and contractual terms and conditions which heavily favour the organization rather than the coaches. These extra costs may be accounted for in the differing rates coaches will have for corporate companies.

For Access to Work funding and self-funded coaching, fees can generally be anywhere between £100 and £250 per session. According to Cowman (2024), the average price for general coaching in the UK is £199 per hour. Corporate fees can be more like £250–£500 per hour. For more specifics for Europe and worldwide, visit www.lir.coach/coach-rates-and-prices-2024-in-the-uk-europe-and-worldwide.

Whether coaches offer a session rate or a package rate for a number of sessions, most will expect fees to be paid upfront or in instalments in advance of the coaching.

Frequency

Standard coaching (executive, leadership, performance coaching, etc.) is usually undertaken on a monthly basis and sometimes fortnightly. ADHD coaching tends to be more frequent in order to keep the momentum going and to get the most impact. It is common for many ADHD coaches to suggest weekly coaching for new clients for one to two months and fortnightly thereafter.

Considering Brown's Executive Function model (2013), more frequent sessions support our working memory and ability to activate and focus on actions we commit to. It also means there is less time to monitor actions before reporting back, which can make it easier for us to engage in process-driven work.

Given we are sprinters rather than marathon runners, it can be helpful to design your coaching like a sprint rather than a seemingly never-ending marathon! Asking for regular review points is an effective way to ensure momentum. Each review point might look at progress made and expectations of where you might like to get to by a certain point in time.

By continually planning for the end in mind, the coaching can feel purposeful and pacey even with the non-linear nature of self-development and our often fabulously creative way of thinking!

GETTING THE MOST OUT OF YOUR COACHING EXPERIENCE

Contracting to find clarity at the beginning of your work together, and at the beginning of sessions (as well as review points through-out the sessions) will help to ensure that you are getting the most out of your coaching. If terms are not agreed and expectations are not aligned, the propensity for you or your coach to end up in drama with each other increases. Coaching needs to be a winning experience where you feel nurtured and learn to nurture yourself, are vulnerable and honest, and learn to be assertive by challenging yourself and others.

As explored in this book, we may not be in touch with what we need and how we feel, which can make speaking up for ourselves in coaching more challenging. This is why regular check-ins about what's working and what isn't are crucial.

Contracting: Getting clear on expectations and making agreements

Part of contracting is getting clear on the desired change. It's very common for prospective coach clients to want tips, tricks, and tools to fix their ADHD so they can 'function normally'. Bottom lining what can change and what might need to be accepted is a challenging conversation, but it's a conversation worth having.

Another part of the contracting process involves setting clear expectations about the commitment required from both you and your coach. A coach will need to be clear about what service and time they are offering. If you are expecting support in between sessions but the coach only provides support during the sessions themselves, this needs to be clear from the start.

Your commitment as a coaching client

Equally important is the commitment required from you. Coaching is generally forward focused, and towards the end of a session it will involve a degree of action from you. This could be being clear on what you might do differently as a result of shifts or insights gleaned in the main part of the session. We frame 'actions' as 'experiments' in ADHD coaching, which helps you to play with how you might activate (take action) on your new thinking. Often, this could be taking time to process information in a way that works for you. This may involve a few experiments as it requires pausing as well as knowing how you process best!

An ADHD coach is *not* an accountability partner (even though it's common for ADHDers to ask for this). A good coach will invite you to reflect on what your wins are compared to what you thought about in the previous session. If you struggle to remember what you committed to this can then inform the actioning for the next session. An example question that a coach might ask here is, 'How can you anchor what you want to retain from this session?'

It is your responsibility to trial ways to remember your 'experiments' outside the coaching sessions, but it is the coach's responsibility to ensure that time is spent exploring past actioning in order to ensure that change and value happen as a result of the coaching process over time.

Sometimes we simply cannot commit to the coaching process. This could be because the level of overwhelm, survival, burnout, or stress is too high in our lives. In this instance, it's a clear indication that coaching is not the best form of support for you at this time. A good coach will be enquiring about your system in the discovery call and/or intake form and will be partnering with you to assess whether coaching is an appropriate support for you.

WHAT IF COACHING ISN'T RIGHT FOR YOU RIGHT NOW?

Let's look at some key things to consider when assessing if ADHD coaching is right for you now.

Assessing readiness for coaching

1. **Self-readiness:** One of the primary considerations is how ready you feel to engage in the coaching process. Coaching requires a level of self-awareness and willingness to

explore personal challenges and growth areas. If you're feeling overwhelmed or resistant to self-exploration, it might be worth considering if this is the right time for coaching.

2. **Ability to engage actively:** Effective coaching requires active participation. You need to be able to engage with your coach, set some intentions, and be willing to try new ways of being and doing. If you find yourself struggling to participate actively due to emotional, mental, or physical reasons, it may be beneficial to address these barriers first.

Considering other factors

1. **Co-occurring mental health challenges:** If you are experiencing significant mental health issues such as severe depression, anxiety, or other psychological challenges, these may need to be well managed before embarking on coaching. In some cases, therapy might be a more appropriate first step to stabilize emotional and psychological well-being. If this is the case, we strongly recommend seeking out a neuro-affirming therapist. The easiest way to tell if they are suitable is to check out what they say about ADHD or neurodiversity on their website; if they don't mention it, ask them upfront – this should give you a good sense of whether they feel right or not.

2. **Systemic changes:** Sometimes, changes in your personal or professional life may make it difficult to continue with coaching or to start in the first place. Significant life events

or stressors can affect your capacity to focus on coaching and its forward motion. It's important to reassess your priorities and possibly pause coaching until your situation stabilizes. This is something that your coach should be open about and willing to explore; they should be explicit about this in the discovery call.

Troubleshooting coaching challenges

1. **Struggling with experimentation and action:** If you find yourself struggling to take action between sessions, it might not necessarily mean that coaching isn't right for you, but perhaps that the approach or the dynamic with the coach needs adjustment. A coach should help you tailor action steps that are realistic and manageable. If actions feel too daunting, discuss scaling back or adjusting these with your coach.

2. **Coach-client dynamic:** Sometimes, the issue might be with the coach-client fit rather than coaching itself. It's vital to feel understood and supported by your coach. If the relationship feels off, consider discussing this with your coach or potentially looking for a new coach who better aligns with your needs.

Alternatives to coaching

1. **Therapy:** For deeper psychological issues or when you need to process past traumas or mental health challenges,

therapy might be more suitable. Therapists can work with you on healing and provide a different form of support that is more introspective and less forward-facing than coaching.

2. **Support groups:** Sometimes, being part of a community facing similar challenges can provide support and insight in ways that one-on-one coaching might not. Support groups for ADHDers can offer camaraderie, understanding, and shared strategies, without the commitment of personal coaching.

3. **Educational workshops and seminars:** If you're not ready for the ongoing commitment of coaching, attending ADHD-related workshops or seminars can provide information and strategies in a less intensive format. This can be a good way to build knowledge and prepare for coaching later on.

Deciding not to engage in coaching at this time doesn't mean closing the door on it forever. It's about choosing the right support at the right time. Reflecting on your current needs, life circumstances, and mental health can help you make an informed decision that best supports your journey with ADHD.

A highly experienced ICF coach, coach mentor and supervisor, Yvette Elcock, helpfully summarizes what to think about if you are looking to end coaching:

When I sense that a coaching relationship might be veering off course or undergoing a shift in some way, my immediate response is to bring it up openly at the start of the next session. Transparency is key in these discussions. It enables both me and my client to openly reassess our alignment and dedication to the goals we set at the beginning of our contract to work together. I cannot stress enough the importance of revisiting the initial agreements, which act as a safety net for both parties. These documents clearly outline our expectations and boundaries, helping us stay anchored to our core objectives and address any deviations head on.

Effective communication is the cornerstone of any successful coaching engagement – it builds towards psychological safety. In my experience, a breakdown in this area is often the root of ineffectiveness. As a coach, I strive to be highly attuned to the subtle cues and communication patterns of my clients. It's not just about being efficient with our time; it's about being truly responsive to the needs that the client presents. This adaptability ensures that the coaching sessions are more than following a set agenda; they are genuinely tailored to foster the growth of the client.

Ethical practice is non-negotiable in coaching. If a coaching dynamic is struggling, it might be necessary for a coach to seek guidance from a supervisor or an ethics committee. These resources can provide invaluable perspectives, ensuring that the coaching remains professional and in the best interest of the coachee. Maintaining the integrity of the coaching process sometimes means making difficult decisions about the continuation of the relationship.

Ending a coaching relationship effectively is as crucial as managing its ongoing dynamics. When it's time to conclude our sessions, I refer back to our initial agreements to ensure that all expectations have been addressed and that the conclusion of our relationship is mutually understood and respectful. If there are unresolved issues, I find it beneficial to involve a neutral third party, such as a mentor or an ally, to provide an outside perspective and facilitate a constructive end to the coaching. This approach helps ensure that the closure is handled with as much care and professionalism as the coaching itself and the opportunity for learning and growth stays present to the end.

As a coach, I view every challenge as a catalyst for growth, for both myself and the people I coach. When facing obstacles, I approach them with honesty, a steadfast commitment to ethics, and an unwavering focus on effective communication. This reflection embodies my coaching philosophy that every difficulty presents an opportunity for development.

YVETTE ELCOCK, ICF COACH AND COACH MENTOR

Here are some refined points to consider if you feel that your ADHD coaching isn't going as expected, along with example actions to help you navigate the situation effectively:

Evaluate your progress: Reflect on the goals and objectives you established at the beginning. Are you closer to achieving them, or do they seem just as distant? This can help determine if the issue is the coaching process or perhaps unrealistic expectations. *Action:* Ask yourself, 'Have I made progress on my specific goals, or am I facing the same challenges as when I started?'

Communicate openly: Honest communication can resolve many issues. If something isn't working, discussing it openly can lead to adjustments that might improve the situation. *Action:* Initiate a conversation with your coach with the question, 'Can we review the coaching methods to see if there might be a better approach to suit my needs?'

Assess the fit: The compatibility between coach and client is crucial for success. If your coach's style isn't a good match for you, it might be time to consider other options. *Action:* Reflect and ask yourself, 'Do I feel understood and supported by my coach, or is there a mismatch in our communication or methods or perspectives?'

Consider timing and external factors: External pressures or life events can impact your engagement with coaching. Assess if these factors are influencing your experience. *Action:* Evaluate, 'Are there external circumstances that are making it difficult for me to engage fully in the coaching process right now?'

Plan for a constructive ending: If you decide to end the relationship, plan to do so in a way that maintains respect and positivity, ensuring you can part ways amicably. *Action:* Prepare to discuss, 'What have I learned from this experience, and how can we ensure a positive conclusion to our coaching sessions?'

These steps encourage a thoughtful approach to addressing concerns with your coaching experience, fostering a productive dialogue, and meaningful reflection to ensure the best possible outcomes.

It is important to remember that speaking up, feeding back, and even stopping coaching or changing coaches is all part of how we stay winning and honour ourselves and protect our ability to thrive. It is *not* failure and instead is often a huge step in self-advocacy!

Finally, it's often through the process of coaching that you may realize that you need different types of support, such as therapy. This realization can be a significant and empowering outcome, demonstrating the success of coaching in helping individuals understand and articulate their needs, leading to self-validation and proactive decision-making.

LIFE BEYOND COACHING

Unlike therapy, which may extend indefinitely depending on the individual's needs and circumstances, ADHD coaching typically spans a more concise timeframe – often ranging from six to twelve months. This structured timeline underscores the goal of coaching: to prepare you to become self-sufficient, eventually making the coaching relationship unnecessary as you learn to coach yourself.

Core identifiers for sustained self-management

There are five key areas that are crucial for continued self-management once ADHD coaching has concluded:

1. **Character strengths utilization:** Using the VIA Character Strengths framework (Peterson & Seligman, 2004), we don't just introduce strengths, we integrate them into daily life. Recognizing and using personal strengths becomes a vernacular – a way of being. For ADHDers, this approach keeps us engaged with our strengths beyond the coaching sessions, ensuring that they remain relevant and integrated into our lives.

2. **Situational awareness:** We emphasize the importance of considering the Task, Individual, and Environment (TIE) in every action. This method helps tailor strategies that align with personal strengths and situational demands, moving away from the unhelpful mantra of 'try harder' to more effective, personalized actions. Where there are environments involving people and power dynamics, situational awareness needs to be seen through an intersectional lens.

3. **Executive function clarity:** Using Brown's (2013) model of Executive Function, we focus on understanding specific areas like activation, focus, effort, emotion, memory, and action monitoring. This clarity helps identify which aspects of executive functioning are aiding or hindering progress, allowing for targeted improvements. Our current state (which we are not always monitoring) will greatly affect how

well our executive function is working. Our state is often being impacted by environments and tasks.

4. **Understanding personal dramas and wins:** Recognizing when we are in a state of 'drama' versus 'winning' allows for better emotional and task management. This understanding directs us towards strategies that shift from reactive to proactive states. Again, our state of drama or winning will be intimately connected to the environments we are navigating and the relative safety we are experiencing. Being discerning about how different environments empower or disempower can be greatly helped by bringing an intersectional lens to drama and winning.

5. **Emotional granularity:** We encourage the use of tools like the Emotions Wheel (Plutchik, 2001) to enhance emotional awareness. This practice can help you articulate your feelings more precisely, leading to better decision-making and fulfilment of your needs.

Transitioning from coaching

Ending the coaching relationship can be challenging, particularly for those who have not experienced healthy conclusions in other areas of their lives. However, concluding well allows for a greater connection to the broader ADHD or neurodivergent community, which can be vital for continued support and growth.

Reflecting on past coach-client experiences, once coaching concludes, the true challenge – and opportunity – begins: maintaining the progress independently. We agree with Suzy (below) – you don't have to work it out alone – even after ADHD coaching.

I don't do well with being told what to do, and ultimately, the power of ADHD coaching is that I have to work it out for myself, but I don't have to work it out alone.

SUZY JACKSON, THE TECHNICOLOUR PROJECT, ADHD SPECIALIST COACH

Here's how you might navigate life after your coaching sessions:

Joining supportive communities: For many people, finding a supportive community post-coaching is crucial. This could be something like joining or initiating a neurodiversity group at work for continued connection and support.

Embracing open dialogue about ADHD: Coaching often empowers you to regain your voice, prompting you to share your stories more openly. Whether through social media, blogs, or even workplace newsletters, talking about ADHD helps to validate experiences and educate others.

Engaging in group processes: For those who find solace in shared experiences, group coaching can be a transformative next step. It offers a space to connect with others who understand the ADHD journey without the need for lengthy explanations or justifications, fostering a deeper communal healing and learning.

Pursuing further education: With the growth of the ADHD

coaching field, many find their next steps in coach training. At Gold Mind Academy, we've seen numerous past coaching clients enrol, eager to deepen their understanding in community and potentially pivot their careers towards serving the diverse community of ADHDers out there.

These steps are not just about continuing the work started in coaching; they're about thriving in a community and culture that recognizes and celebrates ADHD in all its intersectional lenses and co-occurrences. This transition can be a powerful phase of self-discovery and empowerment, marking a new chapter in understanding and leveraging ADHD in all aspects of life.

SUMMARY

Key takeaways
Choosing a qualified coach:

- The coaching industry is not regulated like the medical field, so it's essential to find a coach with proper training.
- It is important to seek a coach with certified ADHD coach training accredited by major coaching bodies like the ICF, EMCC, or PAAC.
- Credentialled coaches adhere to ethical frameworks that provide a structured and professional approach.
- Accredited training ensures the coach is well equipped to work with ADHD-specific challenges and strengths.

Setting up discovery calls:

- Discovery calls allow you to assess the compatibility with potential coaches.
- Take time to meet different coaches to find the best fit for your needs.
- Ensure that you feel safe and understood during these initial interactions.
- Ask about the coach's approach to ADHD coaching, their personal experience, and client success stories.
- Enquire about their qualifications, training hours, and ongoing professional development.
- Ensure that they have the necessary support systems like supervision or mentor coaching.

Safety and intersectionality:

- It's crucial that the coaching environment welcomes all aspects of your identity.
- Discuss your intersecting identities with potential coaches to ensure that they can hold space for your entire experience.
- A safe coaching relationship is one where you can integrate all parts of your identity.

Funding, fees, and frequency:

- Coaching fees vary widely and may depend on who is funding the sessions.
- Be aware of different rates for self-funded, state-funded, and corporate coaching.
- ADHD coaching often requires more frequent sessions

initially to maintain momentum and impact. Weekly sessions may be suggested for the first few months, transitioning to fortnightly.

- Regular review points help track progress and maintain focus.

Getting the most out of your coaching experience:

- Clear contracting at the beginning and regular check-ins are crucial.
- Understand that coaching requires commitment and active participation from you.
- Coaching is forward-focused and involves actioning insights gained during sessions.

Assessing readiness for coaching:

- Reflect on your readiness and ability to engage actively in the coaching process.
- Consider if there are other support needs, such as therapy, that should be addressed first.
- Evaluate your life circumstances to ensure that coaching is the right step at this time.

Life beyond coaching:

- ADHD coaching typically lasts six to twelve months, aiming to make you self-sufficient.
- Post-coaching, engage with supportive communities and continue reflective practices.

- Maintain progress by applying learned strategies and seeking ongoing support when needed.

REFLECTIVE QUESTIONS

1. What qualities are you looking for in an ADHD coach to feel understood and supported?
2. How might working with a qualified ADHD coach differ from your previous support experiences?
3. What aspects of your intersectional identity do you want your coach to acknowledge and integrate into your coaching sessions?
4. What questions are important for you to ask a potential coach to ensure that they meet your needs?
5. How could the frequency and structure of coaching sessions impact your progress?
6. What are your thoughts on the commitment required for coaching, and how prepared are you to engage actively in the process?
7. How might understanding the funding and fees associated with coaching influence your decision?
8. In what ways do you hope to benefit from setting clear expectations and contracting with your coach?
9. How might regular check-ins and reflective practices enhance your coaching experience?
10. What strategies do you think will help you maintain the progress achieved through coaching once it concludes?

CHAPTER 4

What is the Impact of ADHD Coaching?

> The best thing about coaching has been when I have found myself able to use it beyond the session – sometimes intentionally and sometimes instinctively (like magic!), as part of a new habit.
>
> **LILY EASTWOOD, ASSISTANT DIRECTOR**

Everyone's experience of ADHD is different and what they take from coaching will also vary widely depending on what is going on in their system and where they are in their lives. We have taken some general themes which many of you talk about at the end of working with an ADHD coach.

A change narrative is where you reflect on where you were and where you are now and appreciate the pivotal moments that helped you to get there. Getting clarity on your change narrative helps to evidence your capacity for change and can be an important launch pad into future choices. When finishing with an ADHD coach, a discussion about the impact of being coached and all the reflective work that you have done in between sessions is an important part of creating your change narrative.

Clarity around our ability to change is also an important way of getting unstuck from drama positions both with ourselves and with others. If we find ourselves in 'Persecutor' mode but know that change is possible, 'Persecutor' loses its power, as our thoughts about ourselves and others are less fixed. If we find ourselves in 'Victim' mode but remind ourselves that change is possible, we can become unstuck with the memory of previous self-agency. 'Rescuer' is my personal favourite (particularly for those of us in helping professions with tendencies to rescue). If we remind ourselves that we have changed, then we know it is possible for others to change and that they don't need to be rescued with quick-fix solutions. Instead, they may need honesty or curiosity or love, for example...

Interestingly, when first eliciting experience from ADHD coaching clients about the impact of coaching we found that they were often vague, generic, and incredibly short in comparison to the story of struggle before the coaching. What is the ADHD lens on this?

1. The ADHD brain is wired for interest – struggle and challenge are *interesting* whereas the impact of coaching is *important*.
2. Many were being asked to remember ADHD coaching impact that is not in their 'now'.

The second point is why we decided to time the capturing of

some of these change narratives to our clients' 'now' – that is, in the last five minutes of a closing session. You will see this in both Lizzie and Gareth's experiences.

We will start with Gareth's metaphoric change narrative from where he was before ADHD coaching to where he is now:

Walking through a jungle with a Swiss Army knife is not an ideal situation. You would feel unprepared, overwhelmed, unsure how you would get through the thick branches and after a short while you'd probably just give up. This is how I felt every day. Every single day. My brain represents a Mr Messy type figure – you can visualize that, the unorganized lack of pattern type, of shape, that forms Roger Hargreaves's character from Mr Men. It's chaotic, hectic, and it seems as if there is no structure but he still manages to crack a smile or a frown with his single pencil lined mouth and two dots for eyes. Now imagine Mr Messy – with a frown – trying to move through the jungle with a Swiss Army knife. This was me before coaching.

So what did I want from coaching? I wanted my brain to feel organized, have structure, recognize what a 'normal pattern' feels like. I've never ever wanted to be like everyone else but if I could just have a little bit of 'normal' – especially when it came to work – I wanted that! What I got – or what I get – went beyond that. Yes, in a way, I got organized, I got structure, and I started to see the patterns and forms I needed. But, the Mr Messy brain didn't straighten out. The chaotic and hectic sketched lines didn't turn into the sharp right angles of Mr Strong or the smooth completeness of Mr Happy.

The overwhelming vastness of the thick jungle didn't all of a sudden fall away and show me the path through – I got confident in the power of realization, acknowledgement, and self-compassion. I was exactly where I needed to be all along. My brain is still Mr Messy, but now it loves being Mr Messy, because when the single line pencil mouth is frowning it takes The Pause; it accepts, acknowledges the system it's in, and knows that it will be okay. I realize I have a choice and paired with self-compassion that's the most powerful thing we have. Then I work through the models I've learned in coaching to strategize my next move – the choices I have. Instead of my brain thinking, 'I should do this, or I should do that', I change the narrative to 'I could do this, or I could do that' and this has been massive for me and the way I perceive the world and the systems I operate in.

I still have the Mr Messy brain – but now it's chilling in the jungle in a hammock, using the trees instead of trying to hack them down. And, I'm surrounded by my Mr Strong and Mr Happy but they represent the tools I have in the forms of the models and strategies I've learned from my coaching experience.

GARETH DAKIN

In Gareth's visualization of change, we can see some common themes. He acknowledges the chaos, uncertainty, and exhaustion of survival. He admits that when he first came to coaching, he was looking for order and to be 'straightened out' or fixed. This is very common for us to want this as we can be in loops of negative self-talk, and are desperate to fix ourselves. He then goes on to say he did get patterns and structure and certainty but he didn't straighten out and instead it became clear that he was exactly where he was meant to be all along. He talks about the importance of pausing to choose and how he has gone from pressure and expectation ('shoulds'), which don't work well for the interest-wired brain, to possibility and opportunity, which are interest-generating.

We will now explore how one-to-one coaching meets the needs of certainty, clarity, and choice for others. ADHD coaching may be the very start of being in a community with another ADHDer. We end this chapter by exploring and celebrating the power of being in the wider community beyond ADHD coaching.

CERTAINTY

In a similar way to Gareth, Nikki also acknowledges that certainty around challenges can lead to significant action:

> Throughout the year of ADHD coaching, I learned so much about my own ADHD and worked through many challenges. I made adjustments to my home environment to better suit my needs, adapted my work habits, and felt more empowered to advocate for myself. Additionally, I had a supportive

environment to navigate and process the emotions that came with receiving a late diagnosis.

NIKKI HARDY, ADHD CAREER COACH

Certainty around our challenges helps us to bust the shame and become interested. Once we are interested, we take action, as we can see above. In order to feel less judgemental about our challenges, we also need to pay attention to strengths. It's the combination of both that leads to self-compassion, as Lynne acknowledges:

I have developed a much greater understanding of myself. I've been able to notice and appreciate my strengths and develop a more self-compassionate and resourceful inner narrative when it comes to some of the organizational and memory challenges that I will always have due to how my brain is wired.

LYNNE TAPPER, NEURODIVERSITY COACH

Clients often talk about going from feeling awkward and resistant talking about their strengths to a natural fluency – a bit like learning a language:

> I went from naming one strength about me and not really believing it, to thinking I could be any one of these strengths actually.
>
> ANONYMOUS

Once we engage with strengths and become certain that we have them, there can also be a shift from effort to ease:

> Before ADHD coaching, I knew I had strengths but my connection to them was inconsistent to say the least. I could leverage my strengths in service of others but far less in service of myself. So I could only access them when doing things for others and doing more and more and more. Also, strengths were lumped into 'being strong' and making more and more effort.
>
> After coaching, my strengths feel much more nuanced. It's no longer about effort and grind; it's about taking care how I use my energy and strengths. Now, I can separate my strengths out and work out which ones are at play and which ones I need to lean into. My strengths feel more embedded and more intrinsic and my awareness of them is continuing to grow from a place of knowing I have them, rather than hoping I have them.
>
> LIZZIE BENTLEY BOWERS, EXECUTIVE COACH
> AND ADHD SPECIALIST COACH

Lizzie describes the shift from hoping to knowing (certainty) around her strengths and the nuance of them. When we get certainty about our differences and appreciate our strengths, we can let go of ableism and ignorance which affect how we show up for ourselves and others. Here, Thor talks about how coaching helped him move away from ignorance and judgement of himself and break down deeply held beliefs:

Once upon a time, I was one of those parents who believed that ADHD was just an excuse, down to poor parenting, but neurodiversity was closer to me than I ever realized.

Knowing that my eldest was definitely different, like myself, I still fell into the social expectation trap and shamed her before getting her a diagnosis when she was 18 years old, which came after years of struggle.

It is thanks to my children's diagnosis that I came out of this ignorant phase and identified the patterns I was displaying myself. But knowing that I have ADHD only allowed me to understand myself better up to a certain point.

Coaching has helped me understand that my difference is not a bad thing, and it has given me a voice that I felt I was never able to express.

It was through coaching that I was able to reframe my life, that had been filled with shame and constantly punishing myself. It helped me pick up all those different puzzle pieces that I was able to collect by myself and put them together, piece by piece. Coaching is all about breaking down walls and beliefs...

THOR REINHARDT, I AM THOR

In Thor's piece we can see how transformative coaching can be in healing ourselves. Getting certainty with this ADHD lens takes constant reflection and review. This is an important habit that coaching helps us to establish for our ongoing growth.

One of the biggest things I've taken from coaching is learning to pause in situations that I find challenging and consider what's happening through an ADHD lens. I'm learning to forgive myself for perceived failures, to be kinder to myself when I'm frustrated, and lean into just being myself.

For the first time in my life, I'm setting boundaries, putting my needs first, and focusing on what's important to me.

ALLIE WARREN, ADHD COACH AND WORKPLACE CONSULTANT

In Allie's example, we can see how pausing has led her to consider what her needs are and has given her a chance to put in boundaries to protect those needs. Pausing helps us to check in with what is okay and not okay for us. In order to do this, we need to learn how to reconnect and pay attention to bodily sensations, thoughts, and feelings. By reconnecting to ourselves, we get clarity.

CLARITY

When we learn to pause in a structured way using our ADHD lens, we find we can navigate complex situations where we may previously have experienced confusion. Here, Lizzie Bentley Bowers talks about how coaching helped her to speak up in an empowered way for her son's needs at school:

Because of the way that I was coached, I had an empowered knowledge about ADHD. I could articulate what I was observing and what my son needed. There were times when I was able to say, 'I don't believe my son's teachers fully understand the executive functions that are impacted because of his ADHD, for these reasons...' That is just a world away from grappling desperately for words to use. I think the coaching helped with my expectations of the school. I felt confident challenging their terms of reference. I remembered coaching sessions helping me prepare for parents' evenings where I would hear, 'They are not very focused' or, 'They are easily distracted' and I could challenge it in a very adult way and feel really proud of that.

There are many invitations to be pulled into the Drama Triangle when navigating your child's education. And there is this strong pull to be the 'good girl'; there was also a strong pull to be a 'good parent', not a 'difficult parent', but coaching helped me to challenge and manage that. It helped me to trust myself and my knowledge that the system needed to do better by the boys, and helped me build my resilience to challenge again and again... ADHD coaching helped me think about my strengths – what strengths I needed to lean into, and what strengths I needed to build on. It would have been really easy to feel on the back foot and in deficit when dealing with the school, but concentrating on my strengths made me start 'in adult' and stay there, and I am really proud of that.

LIZZIE BENTLEY BOWERS, EXECUTIVE COACH AND ADHD SPECIALIST COACH

Lizzie talks about the propensity to be pulled into drama by normative systems that provide little understanding or flexibility and were expecting her to act a certain way. She is clear that the language and depth of understanding she discovered through coaching – along with challenging old narratives and a focus on strengths – helped her to resist the pull. What has often been a barrier to healthy boundaries is the belief that we are the problem, when in fact other people and our environments are often playing a part. This leads to pedestalling other people and their opinions, which get in the way of us hearing ourselves, what we think, feel, and need. Here, Lizzie talks about how coaching has given her the clarity to figure out what is hers and what isn't in relation to others:

Before ADHD specialist coaching, I cared too much about what other people thought – even that phrase 'I cared too much' was me internalizing other people's criticism. I had to hide the fact that I cared too much because I was ashamed and was repeatedly getting the message that I shouldn't care. I think that message was well intentioned but unhelpful.

After coaching, I do still care what other people think but it is much healthier. I know now that it is not on me to keep trying if my efforts aren't landing and when I am uncertain about people's views of me, I am able to slow that down and work out what is mine and what is theirs and not take all the responsibility. After coaching, I can recognize my rejection sensitivity and I can wait it out or help it out. I ruminate a lot less and can come back to the present much more quickly and easily than I could before coaching.

LIZZIE BENTLEY BOWERS, EXECUTIVE COACH
AND ADHD SPECIALIST COACH

Once we are helped to bring our attention inwards and feel safe enough to bring more of ourselves into the coaching space, we can reflect on situations we find really uncomfortable and work out what we need.

Once we get clarity on our needs in different situations we can get clear on things we may have been tolerating and we can start to make changes in how we communicate our needs and hear the needs of others. Here is an account of how ADHD coaching transformed experience and performance at work:

Through my coaching I began to unpick my needs and started advocating for myself at work to have those needs met. The first step was realizing that I actually have needs and that's okay. Quite often, these are pretty basic, but they are too easy to overlook: regular breaks, clear and direct feedback on my work, and reasonable deadlines so I could source support for more challenging tasks – to name a few.

Through coaching, I was able to start recognizing my strengths and building my self-esteem. I was finally able to disentangle myself (and my ADHD) from the task I was doing and my working environment to get a nuanced understanding of situational variability. This really helped me recognize that I was comfortable with constructive feedback as long as it was clear and given directly to me (rather than via other colleagues who happened to sit near my line manager in a different office to me). It took me a few attempts and some difficult conversations with my line manager to give her direct and quite challenging feedback, but I explained to her that I needed clear and direct communication, choice and agency over my work, and psychological safety. Throughout this process there were tears from both of us, especially when she asked why I wasn't feeling psychologically safe and I said I had given this feedback before and nothing had changed. Eventually I felt heard as she made some changes to my working environment. It was an incredible feeling of relief. I could start to feel more like myself.

ANONYMOUS

Here, the client's ability to nuance that she could welcome feedback if it was done from a place of winning (rather than drama) helped her realize that she did not have to take responsibility for what she had been struggling with but it was her responsibility to feed it back and speak up. The client talks about the big emotional effort it took to speak up but that it was incredibly relieving when she did. Just as others have mentioned how wins lead to more wins, brave challenging can lead to more brave challenging once we realize we can survive it and things can be better.

When we do begin to discover our differences, there is an overwhelming need for understanding and connection from those closest to us, and people's reactions hold huge meaning and power. If we don't get the understanding and acceptance we want, we can flood with disappointment and rejection and be in a state of emotional overwhelm, which can often lead to arguments or withdrawal. The feelings of isolation, loneliness, and shame can actually shut down our prefrontal cortex, making functioning much harder (Cacioppo & Hawkley, 2009; Capodieci, Crisci, & Mammarella, 2019).

Sometimes clarity on our needs can help us take more responsibility for how we have been and still can be! Here, a client talks about how in gifting her relationship more time, she is able to see her own patterns and take positive action:

When I started coaching, my relationship with my partner had been deteriorating since my daughter was born and was on the verge of ending. We were constantly in crisis, with regular arguments that triggered both of us, but they really ramped up my rejection sensitivity.

Before I started to make time and space for 'us' our communication was very limited as I would often work after my daughter went to sleep and, even if I didn't, we were exhausted or overwhelmed with chores and so on, and not in the mood to hold space for each other. We also made a lot of assumptions about why one of us was behaving a certain way.

Through my coaching sessions, I learned how to recognize 'drama' and how to make small changes to coach myself out of it and move into 'thrive'.

I regularly now take a morning off work while my daughter is at school so my partner and I can have brunch together and reconnect. This is a good time of the day for both of us; our energy levels are good and it is dedicated time when we are not also trying to parent, keep the house in order, or work. I have learned much more to listen and ask questions about how my partner is feeling rather than jump to solutions (even if they jump into my head!). This has helped us to rebuild our relationship so that it is now much stronger as we both now have a safer place to talk about our feelings, feel heard, and support each other.

ANONYMOUS

What we see in all the experiences above is that clarity has helped the person to become interested in situations that had previously been important but complex, overwhelming, shame-inducing, or uncomfortable. By getting interested and leaning in, we find choice and freedom.

CHOICE

When we work with interest rather than things we should do, we find it easier to take action because we are taking action by choice.

> I've been coached so much in the past and it's very transactional; 'let's get you from A to B'. There's a little bit of exploring and asking what you have tried in the past and the GROW model, which is useful, but nine times out of ten when I get to the 'Will' bit of GROW, in terms of these are my actions, I never do them! I feel I should do them and I say I will do them, but they never stick.
>
> Whereas in ADHD coaching, it's not transactional, it's going down a few layers and connecting to my feelings and going there. In traditional coaching, the coach's fragility around holding feelings often gets in the way. They are like, 'Oh, you're crying, have some tissues' and then they run away. It's as if they can't go there because they haven't accepted their own emotions and feelings and done the journey with themselves. ADHD coaching is really powerful because we connect to our importance and then it makes

me figure out my next steps in a way that feels as if I want to take action – and I generally do!

MINESH SIYANI, ADHD SPECIALIST COACH AND
LEARNING AND DEVELOPMENT LEAD

Suzy Jackson similarly talks about a freedom in figuring things out their way without feeling there was an unspoken 'right' way:

Traditional coaching often felt like gaslighting to me. I guess because some of the things I'd come up with sounded kind of weird, or off-kilter, or they'd observe things like my lack of eye contact, or tell me what they thought I'd said – which was usually not what I'd said, but also, why are you telling me what I just told you? Who's that helping?

I've found a real authenticity in having ADHD coaching, unlike anything else I've ever experienced. And part of that is definitely the coach, but the other part, the big crucial part, is the coaching. The practice being rooted in how 'my' totally unique and individual brain works, and there really not being any rules of right or wrong, but an open invitation for me to work out what I need, what I want – it's freeing.

SUZY JACKSON, THE TECHNICOLOUR PROJECT,
ADHD SPECIALIST COACH

Choice and freedom can help us to take action or speak up in ways we never thought we would be able to do:

> I've spent decades making myself small as a way of protecting myself and now I've found my voice again, and I'm sharing my thoughts and emotions with others without feeling the intense anxiety that's been present for so long.
>
> ALLIE WARREN, ADHD COACH AND WORKPLACE CONSULTANT

Thor similarly talks about how coaching means he knows how to hack down or free himself from the walls he has been building for decades:

> My journey has allowed me to speak out when I was not able to before. Understanding my ADHD with the help of coaching is allowing me to live the life I was always meant to live. For me, this has resulted in some life-changing decisions that I would have never dared to take in my 'previous life', before my ADHD diagnosis.
>
> It doesn't quite work the way it does in the movies, where I can call my coach/therapist any time I want, when I am struggling. In reality, the coaching that I have had over the last few years now has equipped me with becoming better at breaking down pieces of that wall that I had built up over four decades by myself.

Coaching has equipped me with techniques that I am able to rely on during those dark and tough moments, to remember something positive about myself that seems to 'magically' help me keep going. It's like a piece of that wall just cracked and a huge block of it just blew off.

Coaching has allowed me to understand a fundamental thing – it is not me. I am not a problem.

THOR REINHARDT, I AM THOR

It may seem here that Thor is saying he doesn't get to choose to access support whenever he wants. Instead, coaching has equipped him with the ability to coach himself. What we want and what we need are often very different things!

By continually coaching ourselves to keep hacking off the survival bricks, as Thor says, or the masks we have built up, we often find unexpected buried gold: who we always were but may have temporarily 'lost'.

Right now, I'm the healthiest I've ever been and have a lot more joy in my life. I have rediscovered my sense of humour and my sense of fun that were buried under my mask for so long. And I have learned to love and appreciate my whole self with all of my strengths and all of my ADHD traits – all of my characteristics – so that I am more resilient and emotionally regulated than ever before.

I've also realized that I can be my own role model – I don't need to see others who look and are like me doing the type of job I do – I can be that person for someone else! And I can tell you that my team talks a *lot* more openly about neurodivergence and has higher declarations than many others in my organization, and I think that is wonderful!

ANONYMOUS

When we really see our true selves in all our strengths and challenges, we stop looking for heroes and parents and realize we are the leaders we needed all along. As we can see in the example above, when this happens, everyone around us benefits.

THE POWER OF COMMUNITY

As Cathy Rashidian (2021), ADHD coach and facilitator, has said, 'Don't do ADHD alone.' No true leader is an island. After hiding ourselves away for so long, some of us may need constant reminding of our need for connection and teamwork.

One-to-one ADHD coaching can be the start in breaking down the isolation and shame but there comes a point where being in a wider community with affirming ADHDers can go beyond coaching. Here, Pippa Simou talks about the power of doing ADHD training:

Acceptance of our differences, leaning into them rather than fighting them, is crucial to living well with ADHD. I thought I was accepting of my ADHD but I recently completed some training with Katie and Alex at the Gold Mind Academy which was so valuable to me as it gave me space and time to reflect on the impact of ADHD in my own life. They gave me an opportunity to come to terms with what 'was'– the old stories, the interrupted reaching out – and to recognize the strengths that I showed then, and how those and new strengths can serve me now. I was able to positively reframe my narrative, which has been so helpful to me personally and in my work as a coach. As a result of the training I am even more my authentic self, I am at peace with who 'she' actually is, and I love 'her' more than ever before. The training was a rich experience. Being in a learning environment so suited to my brain, alongside other people in a similar situation, allowed my self-acceptance to grow, which is a precious thing. We all have a need for connection, and connecting with other ADHD folk is such a dynamic, funny, compassionate space to be in, and often the 'best medicine'.

PIPPA SIMOU, ADHD INFORMED COACH

And finally, the allies! It is not solely for us to undertake the work to understand. Here, Yvette Elcock discusses the profound impact of the ADHD training she undertook to understand a neurodivergent family member and the impact on their relationship:

Interacting with an ADHD family member has been a profound journey of learning and adaptation. At the start, I didn't fully grasp the depth of how our neurological differences affected our daily interactions and emotional connections. For instance, the day I decided to organize a room was an eye-opening experience. I had created piles of material to organize and thought I had created order, but when my family member saw it, the sheer amount of organized chaos brought tears. This was more than just clutter; it was a clear sign that our perceptions and ways of processing were fundamentally different.

I have learned the value of patience and the importance of recognizing non-verbal cues. A lower or inconsistent level of eye contact during a discussion doesn't mean a lack of engagement; rather it means, as I now know through discussion, thinking. Learning to interpret these differences correctly has been crucial. It's about understanding that 'different' doesn't mean 'less' and that adjusting my perceptions and reactions can lead to a more harmonious relationship and environment.

Moreover, the experience has been reciprocal. As much as I've learned to adjust my methods and expectations, there has also been a significant effort to meet me halfway. This mutual adaptation has been key to strengthening our relationship. We've learned to discuss our differences openly and to anticipate and accommodate each other's needs, which has minimized misunderstandings and conflicts.

It has taught me that caring effectively involves more than good intentions; it requires well-informed interventions and contributions, actionable understanding and exploration of impact, and the willingness to adapt one's behaviours and expectations. Whether in personal relationships or professional settings, embracing and adapting to neurological differences enriches interactions and fosters genuine connections.

YVETTE ELCOCK, ICF COACH AND COACH MENTOR

ADHD coaching can help us find our voices and advocate for others. Our experience of wider advocacy is as trainers of leaders and managers in organizations. Having been both a manager and an employee who didn't know about her neurodivergence or that of her employees, Katie certainly wishes she had had the training she is now able to provide now she understands herself and feels safer to be vulnerable and model leading with vulnerability to others. Here are some examples of impact as a result of this vulnerability from a recent training event in London:

I appreciate Katie's vulnerability and lived experience. I found myself highly engaged throughout. This training has helped me to reflect on my own behaviours and how that impacts those around me, particularly those who are neurodivergent.

It's provided me with valuable management tools that enable me and my team to be in the Winning Triangle.

GEM AISTON-REEVE, HEAD OF DIGITAL MARKETING

The Neurodiversity Deep Dive has provided an engaging space to learn, reflect, and unpack vulnerability in a supportive environment. I feel better equipped with tools and techniques to work on my assumptions around neurodivergence and to challenge my practice. It has highlighted the importance of naming my own needs and boundaries in order to support the teams I work with.

KELLY MCBRIDE, HEAD OF COMMUNITY ENGAGEMENT

In this way, the ADHD coaching we have had has led us as trainers to positively impact the practice of leaders and managers and so that they can become the allies and the nurturing environment for their neurodivergent employees. And the ripples of positive change continue!

SUMMARY

Key takeaways
Change narrative:

- Reflecting on past experiences and coaching impacts helps to create a narrative of personal change.
- This narrative highlights pivotal moments that contribute to self-awareness and future choices.
- Recognizing one's capacity for change can disrupt negative self-talk and foster self-agency.

Certainty:

- Understanding personal challenges and strengths can lead to significant action and self-advocacy.
- Certainty around one's abilities helps shift from effort to ease and builds self-compassion.
- Acknowledging strengths and challenges reduces shame and fosters personal growth.

Clarity:

- Pausing to reflect helps navigate complex situations and articulate needs effectively.
- Coaching provides clarity on personal strengths, boundaries, and the role of external factors.
- Clear understanding of needs and situational variability enhances self-advocacy and performance.

Choice:

- Coaching equips individuals with the tools to make empowered decisions and advocate for themselves.

- Recognizing personal strengths and abilities enables self-coaching and resilience.
- Making intentional choices based on self-awareness leads to personal growth and fulfilment.

Community:

- One-to-one coaching can be the start of breaking down isolation and shame.
- Engaging with a supportive ADHD community enhances self-acceptance and personal growth.
- Connection with others who understand ADHD provides a dynamic and compassionate support system.

REFLECTIVE QUESTIONS

1. What changes might you hope to see in your life by working with an ADHD coach?
2. How could gaining a better understanding of your strengths and challenges help you take more effective action?
3. What clarity might you gain from pausing to reflect on your experiences with the help of a coach?
4. How might the ability to make more empowered choices influence your daily life and long-term goals?
5. In what ways could developing self-compassion through coaching support your personal and professional growth?

6. How might coaching empower you to better understand and advocate for your needs and strengths?

7. What benefits could you experience from connecting with a supportive ADHD community?

Final Words

As we draw to a close and reflect on our journey through this book, several key themes emerge:

- Empowerment through strengths.
- The importance of professional support.
- Navigating intersectional experiences of normative power systems and how this impacts our ADHD.
- Ongoing self-discovery.
- Tailored strategies are critical components of effective ADHD management.

These themes not only encapsulate the essence of ADHD coaching but also provide a roadmap for individuals seeking to understand and navigate their ADHD more effectively.

FINAL REFLECTIVE QUESTIONS

1. How has your understanding of ADHD evolved through this book, and what new insights have you gained about your own or others' experiences?
2. In what ways do you think ADHD coaching can change your approach to personal and professional challenges?
3. How do your various identities intersect with your experience of ADHD, and how can this awareness influence your approach to seeking support?
4. What steps can you take to ensure that the progress made during coaching continues beyond the formal coaching relationship?
5. How can you leverage community resources and support systems to continue your journey of growth and self-discovery with ADHD?

ADHD coaching offers a transformative approach to understanding and managing ADHD. By focusing on strengths, advocating for professional and ethical support, and recognizing the importance of intersectional identities, we can foster an environment where individuals with ADHD thrive. As you continue to explore and embrace your unique potential, we hope these insights and reflections guide you towards a more empowered and fulfilling experience with your ADHD.

References

Abdelnour, E., Jansen, M. O., & Gold, J. A. (2022). ADHD diagnostic trends: Increased recognition or overdiagnosis? *Missouri Medicine, 119*(5), 467–473.

ADHD UK. (n.d.). The history of ADHD. Retrieved from https://ADHDuk.co.uk/the-history-of-ADHD/#:~:text=2000&text=For%20the%20first%20time%2C%20the,NICE%20formally%20recognizes%20childhood%20ADHD.

American Medical Association. (2016). Disability, medicine, and ethics. *AMA Journal of Ethics.* https://journalofethics.ama-assn.org.

American Psychological Association. (n.d.). Therapy. In *APA Dictionary of Psychology.* Retrieved from https://dictionary.apa.org/therapy.

Arnsten, A. F. (2009). Toward a new understanding of attention-deficit hyperactivity disorder pathophysiology: An important role for prefrontal cortex dysfunction. *CNS Drugs, 23*(Suppl 1), 33–41.

Asasumasu, K. (2000). Coined the term 'neurodivergent'. (No specific publication available.)

Barkley, R. A. (2006). *Attention-Deficit Hyperactivity Disorder: A Handbook for Diagnosis and Treatment* (third edition). New York, NY: Guilford Press.

Barkley, R. A. (2012). *The Important Role of Executive Functioning and Self-Regulation in ADHD.* New York, NY: Guilford Press.

Barkley, R. A. (2015). *Attention-Deficit Hyperactivity Disorder: A Handbook for Diagnosis and Treatment* (fourth edition). New York, NY: Guilford Press.

Barnes, A. (2022). ADHD was never the problem, not knowing was. In *Interview with Funny Women.* Retrieved from https://funnywomen.com/2022/01/11/angela-barnes-reports-on-ADHD-for-the-one-show.

Barrett, L. F. (2017). *How Emotions are Made: The Secret Life of the Brain.* Boston, MA: Houghton Mifflin Harcourt.

Briere, J. & Scott, C. (2014). *Principles of Trauma Therapy: A Guide to Symptoms, Evaluation, and Treatment* (second edition). Los Angeles, CA: Sage Publications.

Brown, B. (2018). *Dare to Lead: Brave Work. Tough Conversations. Whole Hearts.* New York, NY: Random House.

Brown, T. E. (2004). *Attention Deficit Disorder: The Unfocused Mind in Children and Adults.* New Haven, CT: Yale University Press.

Brown, T. E. (2013). *A New Understanding of ADHD in Children and Adults: Executive Function Impairments.* New York, NY: Routledge.

Brown, T. E. (2017). *Outside the Box: Rethinking ADD/ADHD in Children and Adults: A Practical Guide*. Washington, DC: American Psychiatric Association Publishing.

Brown, T. E. (2023). Lifelong ADHD: Rethinking the adult diagnosis. *Journal of Developmental & Behavioral Pediatrics*, 44(2), 112–119.

Cacioppo, J. T. & Hawkley, L. C. (2009). Perceived social isolation and cognition. *Trends in Cognitive Sciences*, 13(10), 447–454.

Capodieci, A., Crisci, G., & Mammarella, I. C. (2019). Does positive illusory bias affect self-concept and loheliness in children with symptoms of ADHD? *Journal of Attention Disorders*, 23(11), 1274–1283.

Choudhury, A. (2021). *Anticipatory inclusion*. Retrieved from www.diversityandability. com/team/atif-choudhury.

Coates, T. (2015). *Between the World and Me*. New York, NY: Spiegel & Grau.

Coker, T. R., Elliott, M. N., Schwebel, D. C., Cuccaro, P., et al. (2016). Racial and ethnic disparities in ADHD diagnosis and treatment. *Pediatrics*, 138(3).

Council of the London Borough of Haringey. (1986). Officially used the term 'ableism.' (No specific publication available.)

Cowman, L. (2024). Coach rates and prices 2024 in the UK, Europe, and worldwide. Retrieved from www.lir.coach/coach-rates-and-prices-2024-in-the-uk-europe-and-worldwide.

Crenshaw, K. (1989). Demarginalizing the intersection of race and sex: A black feminist crltique of antidiscrimination doctrine, feminist theory and antiracist politics. *University of Chicago Legal Forum*, 1989(1), article 8.

Criado Perez, C. (2019). *Invisible Women: Exposing Data Bias in a World Designed for Men*. New York, NY: Abrams Press.

Csíkszentmihályi, M. (1990). *Flow: The Psychology of Optimal Experience*. New York, NY: Harper & Row.

Dethmer, J., Chapman, D., & Klemp, K. (2015). *The 15 Commitments of Conscious Leadership: A New Paradigm for Sustainable Success*. Conscious Leadership Group.

Ditzler, J. (2003). *Your Best Year Yet! Ten Questions for Making the Next Twelve Months Your Most Successful Ever*. New York, NY: Grand Central Publishing.

Dodson, W. W. (2016). Emotional dysregulation and ADHD. CHADD. Retrieved from https://chadd.org/wp-content/uploads/2016/10/ATTN_10_16_EmotionalRegulation.pdf.

Doyle, N. (2020). Neurodiversity at work: A biopsychosocial model and the impact on working adults. *British Medical Bulletin*, 135(1), 108–125.

Doyle, N. (2024). *Neurodiversity at Work: A Biopsychosocial Approach*. London: Inclusion Press.

Doyle, N. & McDowall, A. (2024). *Neurodiversity Coaching: A Psychological Approach to Supporting Neurodivergent Talent and Career Potential*. London: Routledge.

Durkheim, E. (1895). *The Rules of Sociological Method* (S. Lukes, ed.). New York, NY: Free Press. (Original work published in French.)

Faraone, S. V., Asherson, P., Banaschewski, T., Biederman, J., et al. (2015). Attention-deficit/hyperactivity disorder. *Nature Reviews Disease Primers*, 1, 15020.

Friedman, L. A. & Sterling, J. (2019). The role of fatigue in the pathogenesis of burnout among individuals with ADHD: Exploring the neurodiversity paradigm. *Journal of Neurodiversity Studies*, 1(1), 12–24.

Gott, C. (2024, July). ADHD coaching, flow, and hyperfocus [LinkedIn post]. LinkedIn. Retrieved from www.linkedin.com/posts/camerongott_ADHDcoach-flow-hyperfocus-activity-7212142498394107904-xfeY.

Hamilton, P. (1938). *Gas Light*. London: Richmond Theatre.

Hallowell, E. M. (2019). Your ADHD Brain is a Ferrari. Retrieved from https://drhallowell.com/2019/04/05/your-ADHD-brain-is-a-ferrari.

Hallowell, E. M. & Ratey, J. J. (2021). ADHD 2.0: New Science and Essential Strategies for Thriving with Distraction – From Childhood Through Adulthood. New York, NY: Ballantine Books.

Hinshaw, S. P. (2018). The ADHD Explosion: Myths, Medication, Money, and Today's Push for Performance. Oxford: Oxford University Press.

Høglend, P. (2014). Exploration of the patient-therapist relationship in psychotherapy. The American Journal of Psychiatry, 171(10), 1056–1066.

hooks, b. (2000). Feminism is for Everybody: Passionate Politics. Cambridge, MA: South End Press.

International Coaching Federation. (n.d.). What is coaching? Retrieved from https://coachingfederation.org/about#:~:text=What%20is%20Coaching%3F,of%20imagination%2C%20productivity%20and%20leadership.

Joshi, G., Faraone, S. V., Wozniak, J., Tarko, L., et al. (2017). Symptom profile of ADHD in youth with high-functioning autism spectrum disorder: A comparative study in psychiatrically referred populations. Journal of Attention Disorders, 21(9), 846–855.

Karpman, S. (1968). Fairy tales and script drama analysis. Transactional Analysis Bulletin, 7(26), 39–43.

Kessler, R. C., Adler, L., Barkley, R., Biederman, J., et al. (2006). The prevalence and correlates of adult ADHD in the United States: Results from the National Comorbidity Survey Replication. American Journal of Psychiatry, 163(4), 716–723.

Kirby, A. & Smith, T. (2021). Neurodiversity at Work: Drive Innovation, Performance and Productivity with a Neurodiverse Workforce. London: Kogan Page Publishers.

Maslow, A. H. (1943). A theory of human motivation. Psychological Review, 50(4), 370–396. https://doi.org/10.1037/h0054346.

Morgan, P. L., Staff, J., Hillemeier, M. M., Farkas, G., & Maczuga, S. (2013). Racial and ethnic disparities in ADHD diagnosis from kindergarten to eighth grade. Pediatrics, 132(1), 85–93. doi:10.1542/peds.2012-2390.

Nair, V. K., Farah, W., & Boveda, M. (2024). Is neurodiversity a Global Northern White paradigm? Autism. https://doi.org/10.1177/13623613241280835.

Oliver, M. (1983). Social Work with Disabled People. London: Macmillan.

Oliver, M. (1990). The Politics of Disablement. London: Macmillan.

Parush, S., Sohmer, H., Steinberg, A., & Kaitz, M. (2007). Somatosensory function in boys with ADHD and tactile defensiveness. Physiology & Behavior, 90(4), 553–558.

Parton, D. (n.d.). 'Find out who you are and do it on purpose.' Retrieved from www.southernliving.com/author/nellah-bailey-mcgough.

Perry, G. (2017). The Descent of Man. London: Penguin.

Peterson, C. & Seligman, M. E. P. (2004). Character Strengths and Virtues: A Handbook and Classification. New York, NY: Oxford University Press.

Plutchik, R. (2001). The nature of emotions. American Scientist, 89(4), 344–350.

Porges, S. W. (2007). The polyvagal perspective. Biological Psychology, 74(2), 116–143.

Professional Association for ADHD Coaches. (n.d.). What is ADHD coaching? Retrieved from www.paaccoaches.org.

Quinn, P. O. (2005). Gender differences in ADHD. Journal of Clinical Psychology, 61(5), 579–587.

Quinn, P. O. (2005). Treating adolescent girls and women with ADHD: Gender-specific issues. Journal of Clinical Psychology, 61(5), 579–587.

Rashidian, C. (2021). Don't do ADHD alone. Retrieved from www.understood.org/articles/en/working-mom-with-ADHD-feeling-control-over-nothing.

Reeves, A. & Friedman, S. (2024). *Born to Rule: The Making and Remaking of the British Elite.* Cambridge, MA: Harvard University Press.

Robbins, T. (2021). *The 6 human needs from Tony Robbins that shape our life.* Retrieved from www.tonyrobbins.com.

Shapiro, F. (2001). *Eye Movement Desensitization and Reprocessing (EMDR): Basic Principles, Protocols, and Procedures* (second edition). New York, NY: Guilford Press.

Singer, J. (1998). *Odd People In: The Birth of Community Amongst People on the Autistic Spectrum: A Personal Exploration of a New Social Movement Based on Neurological Diversity* (Honours thesis). University of Technology, Sydney.

van der Kolk, B. (2014). *The Body Keeps the Score: Brain, Mind, and Body in the Healing of Trauma.* New York, NY: Viking.

VIA Institute on Character. (n.d.). The VIA character strengths survey. VIA Institute on Character. www.viacharacter.org.

Volkow, N. D., Wang, G. J., Kollins, S. H., Wigal, T. L., *et al.* (2009). Evaluating dopamine reward pathway in ADHD: Clinical implications. *Journal of the American Medical Association, 302*(10), 1084–1091.

Walby, S. (1990). *Theorizing Patriarchy.* Oxford: Blackwell.

Walker, N. (2014). Neurodiversity: Some basic terms & definitions. *Neurocosmopolitanism.* Retrieved from http://neurocosmopolitanism.com/neurodiversity-some-basic-terms-definitions.

Warner, M. (1993). *Fear of a Queer Planet: Queer Politics and Social Theory.* Minneapolis, MN: University of Minnesota Press.

Weber, M. (1946). *From Max Weber: Essays in Sociology.* New York, NY: Oxford University Press.

Wiener, J. & Daniels, T. (2016). Empathy in children with attention deficit hyperactivity disorder (ADHD). *Journal of Child and Family Studies, 25*(4), 1149–1157. doi:10.1007/s10826-015-0309-2.

Wiseman, H. & Tishby, O. (2017). Applying relationship anecdotes paradigm interviews to study client–therapist relationship narratives: Core conflictual relationship theme analyses. *Psychotherapy Research, 27,* 283–299.

Wise, S. J. (2024). *We're All Neurodiverse: How to Build a Neurodiversity-Affirming Future and Challenge Neuronormativity.* London: Jessica Kingsley Publishers.

World Education Services. (n.d.). *Mentoring: Building a relationship for success.* Retrieved from www.wes.org/advisor-blog/mentoring-building-a-relationship-for-success.

Yochman, A., Parush, S., & Ornoy, A. (2004). Responses of preschool children with and without ADHD to sensory events in daily life. *American Journal of Occupational Therapy, 58*(3), 294–302.

Young, S., Adamo, N., Ásgeirsson, H., Brandt, V., *et al.* (2020). Guidance for identification and treatment of individuals with attention deficit/hyperactivity disorder and autism spectrum disorder. *BMC Medicine, 18,* 146.

Zablotsky, B., Bramlett, M. D., & Blumberg, S. J. (2020). The co-occurrence of autism spectrum disorder in children with ADHD. *Journal of Attention Disorders, 24*(1), 94–103. doi:10.1177/1087054717713638.

Zulauf-McCurdy, S. (2023). Underdiagnosed and Undertreated, Young Black Males With ADHD Get Left Behind. KFF Health News. Retrieved from https://kffhealthnews.org/news/article/black-children-ADHD-diagnosis-disparities.